W9-ANR-958

Praise for *Impossible Cure*

"Many of the greatest advances in science and medicine begin as observations that don't fit in. Homeopathy – the 'impossible cure' – is just that sort of challenge. Amy Lansky is a skilled guide to the world of homeopathy, and she dispels much of the mystery surrounding this form of therapy. *Impossible Cure* is a valuable insight for anyone wishing to know more about homeopathy and how it may fit into their search for health."

— LARRY DOSSEY, MD
Executive Editor, Alternative Therapies in Health and Medicine
Author: *Healing Beyond the Body*, *Reinventing Medicine*, and *Healing Words*

"By writing *Impossible Cure*, author Amy Lansky has accomplished a (nearly) impossible task: provide a clear, comprehensible, and compelling exposition of homeopathy. Her autistic son's remarkable response to homeopathic treatment motivated computer scientist Lansky to bring the long-neglected science of homeopathy to public attention. She has succeeded admirably. *Impossible Cure* is timely, informative, and remarkably reader friendly. An excellent, must-read book. Highly recommended!"

— BERNARD RIMLAND, PhD
Director, Autism Research Institute; Founder, Autism Society of America

"The finest general introduction to homeopathy I've yet read...This book should be read by everyone interested in homeopathy, from the rank beginner to the seasoned professional. It has something new in it for everyone."

— JULIAN WINSTON
Editor, *Homeopathy Today*
Author: *The Faces of Homeopathy* and *The Heritage of Homeopathic Literature*

"This book may very well contribute to the transformation of homeopathy from the ugly duckling of medicine to the swan that it deserves to be."

— LIA BELLO, RN, FNP, CCH
Reviewer for *Homeopathy Today*

"A well-written and ultimately inspiring volume... Impossible Cure presents an uncompromising call for a rethinking of conventional medical practices in the U.S."

— **D. PATRICK MILLER**

Fearless Books Review (www.fearlessbooks.com)

"Homeopathy is *the* emerging therapy that offers hope for truly curing chronic disease in a profound way. This book is a comprehensive introduction to the full extent of what homeopathy can do for you. By providing case histories, deep yet understandable explanations of homeopathy (including its relationship to modern medicine), and clear information on what it means to be a homeopathic patient, *Impossible Cure* is an invaluable resource. A perfect book for patients and first-year students of homeopathy."

— **LOUIS KLEIN, RSHOM**

President, Luminos Homeopathic Courses Ltd., Luminos Schools,
and Homeopathic Master Clinicians Course *(www.homeopathycourses.com)*
Author: *Clinical Focus Guide to Homeopathic Remedies* and
Luminos Homeopathic Provings

"Amy Lansky watched in disbelief as homeopathy did the impossible — cured her son, Max, of autism. She delved into the controversial therapy and has become an articulate, passionate advocate for the healing art most physicians continue to dismiss as 'impossible.' Her book is filled with a mother's love and a scientist's skepticism. The result is one of the best introductions to homeopathy I've seen. Two thumbs up for *Impossible Cure: The Promise of Homeopathy*."

— **MICHAEL CASTLEMAN**

Author: *The Healing Herbs, The New Healing Herbs, Nature's Cures, Blended Medicine,* and other consumer health books

"An accessible guide to one of the most mysterious of healing arts."

— **WAYNE B. JONAS, MD**

Director, Samueli Institute

Impossible Cure

THE PROMISE OF HOMEOPATHY

Amy L. Lansky, PhD

With a foreword by Richard Pitt, CCH, RSHom (NA)

R.L. Ranch

Press

Portola Valley, California

Impossible Cure: The Promise of Homeopathy.
Copyright © 2003 by Amy L. Lansky, PhD.

Printed and bound in the United States of America. All rights reserved. No part of this book may be reproduced or transmitted in any form or by any electronic or mechanical means, including photocopying, recording, or by an information storage and retrieval system, without permission from the Publisher — except in the case of brief quotations embodied in reviews and academic papers. For more information, please contact:

R.L.Ranch Press
4119 Alpine Road, Suite A
Portola Valley, California 94028
Tel: 650-851-2927
Fax: 650-851-9095
E-mail: info@impossiblecure.com

Visit our web site:
www.impossiblecure.com
to find out more about homeopathic treatment
and about bulk discount orders of this book.

Although the author and publisher have exhaustively researched all sources to ensure the accuracy and completeness of information contained in this book, we assume no responsibility for errors, inaccuracies, omissions, or any inconsistency herein. Any slights of people, places, or organizations are unintentional.

PUBLISHER'S CATALOGING-IN-PUBLICATION DATA
Lansky, Amy L., 1955–
    Impossible cure : the promise of homeopathy / Amy L.
Lansky ; with a foreword by Richard Pitt.
    p.   cm.
    Includes bibliographical references and index.
    LCCN 2003090295
    ISBN 0-9727514-0-8
    1. Homeopathy.   I. Title.
RX71.L367 2003   615.5'32
                                                    QBI03-200087

SECOND PRINTING, 2004

Interior and cover design by Melanie Haage
Author photo by Jennifer Dungan
Book production by Data Reproductions Corporation
Printed in the United States of America

For Steve, Izaak, and Max

Dare to know
That the source of all miracles
Lies within you.

SPECIAL NOTICE TO THE READER

Although this book discusses the homeopathic method of treatment, including stories of cure using various remedies, it is intended only as a general introduction to homeopathy. It is not meant to give specific recommendations of medical, psychological, or other advice regarding the treatment of particular illnesses. Nor does it make any warranties or guarantees of any sort that any of the information in this book (or in any of the books or material listed under "Suggested Reading" and "Helpful Resources") will produce any particular medical, physical, emotional or other result. This book is not intended to be a replacement for good medical diagnosis and treatment by a licensed physician or for care by a certified health-care practitioner. Readers are strongly cautioned to consult with a licensed health-care professional before utilizing any information in this book, and if they choose to pursue to homeopathic treatment, to do so under the supervision of a licensed physician and a certified homeopath.

Permissions

Special thanks to all of the individuals who allowed me to use their stories of homeopathic healing in this book. Special thanks also go to North Atlantic Books and Homeopathic Educational Services of Berkeley, California, for permission to quote from several of their books. These include *Psyche and Substance*, by Edward C. Whitmont (copyright © 1991 by Edward C. Whitmont, MD); *Divided Legacy, Volume III*, by Harris Livermore Coulter (copyright © 1973 by Harris L. Coulter); and *A Homeopathic Love Story*, by Rima Handley (copyright © 1990 by Rima Handley). North Atlantic Books has given permission to quote from *The Emerging Science of Homeopathy*, by Paolo Bellavite and Andrea Signorini (copyright © 2002 by Paolo Bellavite, MD and Andrea Signorini, MD). I also thank Grove/Atlantic, Inc. for their permission to quote from *The Science of Homeopathy*, by George Vithoulkas (copyright © 1980 by George Vithoulkas). Heartfelt thanks to Julian Winston, for his permission to use numerous quotes from his classic volume on homeopathic history, *The Faces of Homoeopathy*, published by Great Auk Publishing, Tawa, New Zealand (copyright © 1999 by Julian Winston). Julian also has given permission in his capacity as editor of *Homeopathy Today* to use several quotes from that magazine, published by the National Center for Homeopathy, Alexandria, Virginia. Thanks to Rajan Sankaran for permission to quote from his books *The Spirit of Homeopathy* (copyright © 1992 by Dr. Rajan Sankaran) and *The Soul of Remedies* (copyright © 1997 by Dr. Rajan Sankaran). Ian Watson has given permission to use several quotes from his book *A Guide to the Methodologies of Homeopathy* (copyright © 1999 by Ian Watson). Finally, thanks to the publishers of *Alternative Therapies*, *The Scientist*, *Pediatrics*, *The American Homeopath*, and *The Lancet* for permission to quote and discuss papers published in their respective journal publications, including, in some cases, the use of tables. All of the above credits and every other quotation in this book have been duly cited in the text and are accompanied by citation descriptions in the references section at the end of this book.

TABLE OF CONTENTS

FOREWORD

HOMEOPATHY IS ONE OF THE MOST ENIGMATIC OF MEDICAL ARTS. Born out of 18th-century medical and scientific thinking, steeped in a tradition of empirical rationalism, and coming to light at a crucial crossroads in Western thought, homeopathy has never been widely accepted within mainstream medicine. Even though it achieved remarkable popularity in the 19th century, both in Europe and the United States, its very existence challenged the established Newtonian view of the world, one defined by a mechanistic view of the human body.

The founder of homeopathy, Samuel Hahnemann — a chemist, scholar, and physician — was influenced not only by the "new" way of thinking about the body entailed by enlightenment philosophy, but also by a more alchemical view of the world, where the mystery of the hidden meanings, functions, and interconnections of all things needed to be acknowledged. These influences led to the development of his concept of *vital force*, a quality of energy that is both immaterial (cannot be seen) and also all encompassing in its influence over biological function. By no means the first to speak of such phenomena, *qi* being understood by the Chinese for three thousand years and *prana* being recognized by the Indian philosophers for a similar time, Hahnemann integrated this concept into a rational system of medical healing, which was unique in the West. The 15th-century alchemist/physician Paracelsus attempted a similar synthesis, but he never got far beyond the empirical drawing board.

Therefore, even if thinkers could accept the apparent contradictions of the homeopathic law of cure, "Let Likes Be Cured by Likes," when it came to the concept of a vital force permeating and influencing the anatomy and physiology of human organisms, this was too much for most to bear. Two hundred years later, we are faced with the same dilemma, although cracks are continually appearing in the dam of scientific materialism. Homeopathy is but one of the wedges forcing these cracks, its philosophy and position as a legitimate medical art practiced by physicians being a recurring irritation in the attempts to constrain medical doctrine to only that which we can see and control.

There is now a tidal wave of change occurring within the fields of medicine, psychology, physics, and the panoply of healing modalities available, with ample evidence suggesting that people are looking for alternative models of healing, even if they don't know how they work. In many ways, science and medicine are now catching up with what many people already know and have experienced. These things do work. Also, faced with the exploding costs and health complications of conventional medicine, new models of healing are coming to the forefront of people's attention. Homeopathy is one of them.

However, the challenge that homeopaths have always grappled with is how to demystify its approach to healing and help people understand what embarking into homeopathic treatment is all about. While on the surface it seems like Western medicine, with tablets being given as the remedy, the process of homeopathic treatment is a mix of visiting your doctor, psychiatrist, therapist, and a private detective. Part of the confusion seems to be that it is all of these things at the same time. It is hard to categorize into convenient boxes. It is medicine and healing, incorporating mind, body, and soul, physical disease and mental conditioning, fusing energy and matter into an inseparable whole.

How to communicate this amazing science and art? Many books have been written on homeopathy, some good and others not, often attempting to cross the bridge between the esoteric workings of the profession and a more mainstream understanding of its process. However, homeopathy is still not understood by most people, even two hundred years later. Even in more enlightened spheres, anything more than a superficial understanding of homeopathy is hard to find.

In *Impossible Cure*, Amy Lansky is going one step further in enlightening us to the potential of homeopathy and its fascinating history. Her personal experience of finding a homeopathic cure for her son's autism is extraordinary enough. However, she has laid out one of the most complete pictures of homeopathy ever written. The book is extremely well researched, and Lansky has managed to make it accessible to an average reader in a way that will open people's minds about homeopathy. It will also help others already in the health-care field to learn about the potential of homeopathic treatment and to recognize that, in homeopathy, we have one of the most unique and complete systems of medicine available. Like a hidden treasure sitting in a basement for two hundred years, the jewels of homeopathy need to see the light of day. *Impossible Cure* will help do this. It is a superb document, and for those of us who practice and teach homeopathy, it is an exciting development — one that will help homeopathy take its appropriate place in medicine today.

Richard Pitt, CCH, RSHom (NA)
Homeopath and Educator
Director, Pacific Academy of Homeopathy
San Francisco, California
November 2002

PREFACE

TEN YEARS AGO, I WOULD NEVER HAVE IMAGINED MYSELF SITTING here, in an office nestled among the trees behind my home, writing a preface to a book about homeopathy. Back then, in November of 1992, I was caught up in my computer science research work at NASA, trying to play the academic game. Between my family and my job, life was busy and often stressful.

Of course, things can change. As the bumper sticker says, "Life Happens." And nothing is more transformative than a crisis with one's children. Children come first, and if things go wrong for them, the fabric of life can easily unravel. When my son Max started manifesting symptoms of autism, I, like most parents faced with this kind of situation, was caught between two feelings: that things were "fine" and would blow over, or that something was terribly and inexorably wrong. The feelings of dread in my gut told me that the latter was correct.

My husband and I pressed forward as best as we could. I was determined to help Max recover, not just for his sake, but for my own sake and for the rest of my family as well. I was searching for — and open to — a solution. When I read about homeopathy, it somehow struck me as the way. God was certainly watching over us that day and over the course of the next several years, as we all walked the winding road back to health.

It didn't take long for me to realize that my son's miraculous cure from autism was far more revolutionary than any computer program or technological gadgetry. Just as the dot-com revolution hit Silicon Valley, a disenchantment with Silicon Valley hit me. My work in computer science suddenly seemed banal and trivial in comparison to what had happened to Max. I began to study homeopathy myself and soon became enthralled and enchanted. I could not believe that such a marvelous medical science could be so unknown to most people. Eventually, I realized that I had to write a book to let everyone know about it. And I also had to let other parents know that there was hope for their kids too. If one other child could be helped the way Max was, all my efforts would be worthwhile.

Today, after many years of research and writing, studying homeopathy to prepare for my own future practice, and treading political waters in an effort to legalize homeopathic practice in my own state of California (with success!), I realize that the most effective way to let people know about the treasure of homeopathy is to present a firsthand view — not a theoretical convincement. Dear reader, the homeopathic vista is there for you to behold and enjoy if you're willing to travel there and hike its trails and hills and valleys. This book is an attempt to describe its panoramic beauty and potential. It is up to you to take the next step and experience homeopathy for yourself. I hope you will.

Amy L. Lansky, PhD
Portola Valley, California
November 2002

ACKNOWLEDGMENTS

I WON'T SAVE THE BEST FOR LAST. I OWE EVERYTHING TO MY FAMILY — my husband Steve Rubin and my two sons, Izaak and Max Rubin. They are my joy, my shelter in the storm, and the providers of all the support and encouragement anyone could desire.

Outside of this innermost circle are the friends and colleagues who have advised and spirited me on throughout my growth as a homeopath and writer. The most insightful and influential input into this book was provided by my husband Steve, who served as my first and last reader, and by two very dear friends named Richard: Richard Gabriel — poet, author, fellow computer scientist, and awesome lead-guitarist; and Richard Pitt — seeker, teacher, homeopath, and an important voice of responsibility and wisdom in the growing homeopathic world. Invaluable input into this book and its production was also provided by Julian Winston, premier historian of homeopathy; Wenda Brewster O'Reilly, editor of the newest and best translation of the *Organon*; and Maggie Taeger, a friend and fellow student of homeopathy. From the beginning until the end of my journey in writing and producing this book, author Dean Radin provided tips, advice, and leads into the publishing world. Others who read this book in its various stages and provided advice and encouragement include: Sally Ahnger, Jennifer Dungan, Russell Targ, Sandra Martin, Patrick Huyghe, Chris Wellens, Bruce Horn, and, of course, John Melnychuk, our family homeopath who, in many ways, made it all possible. Love and support were also provided by my mother Jeanette Lansky, Laura Hertzfeld, and Bertha Philyaw.

Of course, much of this book is about the firsthand experience of homeopathy. This was made possible by generous input from many wonderful homeopaths and patients who contributed their stories to this book. They did so with the hope that they would be helping others to find healing, so please join me in sending love and thanks their way. Nearly all of these individuals have been participants in an international on-line community devoted to homeopathy, and many of its members have become my teachers and friends.

My own firsthand experience of homeopathy was made possible by those individuals who have been instrumental in healing my son Max and the rest of my family. My family's journey to homeopathy was set in motion by an article in *Mothering* magazine written by Judyth Reichenberg-Ullman. We were then guided to our family homeopath, John Melnychuk, by Joan Kobara. Max's cure was also enabled by his language therapist Donna Dagenais and by osteopath Mark Rosen. My own healing process was facilitated by homeopaths Simon Taffler and Sally Williams.

I learned much of the information in this book from teachers and fellow students of homeopathy. I have studied under the guidance of Misha Norland, Simon Taffler, Sadhna Thakkar, Louis Klein, Jan Scholten, Alize Timmerman, Will Taylor, David Little, Julian Winston, John Melnychuk, Jo Daly, Murray Feldman, Janet Snowdon, Jeremy Sherr, and Rajan Sankaran. My fellow students are too numerous to mention, but special thanks go to Jonathan Pierce, Leslie Platner, Keith Kale, Janet Mandell, Pam Klein, Joy Wilson, Maggie Taeger, and Gini Ellis.

Last but not least are those who have guided and helped me through the formidable book production process. Many thanks to my copy editor Jim Gebbie for a quick and thorough job, and to my talented book designer Melanie Haage, who created a book whose beauty will be appreciated by all. I would also like to thank Marilyn and Tom Ross for their invaluable book on publishing and book promotion, and the folks at Data Reproductions Corporation.

CHAPTER 1

><

HOMEOPATHY REVEALED

"Aude Sapere"
(*"Dare to Know"*)

—SAMUEL HAHNEMANN, MD

Title page epigraph, *The Organon of the Medical Art,* 1810 [Hahnemann]

IT MAY SEEM UNBELIEVABLE, BUT IT'S TRUE. MY SON WAS CURED of an incurable illness with a form of medicine that supposedly contains nothing — at least according to conventional scientific thought. But, as history has repeatedly shown, the accepted scientific and medical wisdom of an era can be wrong.

It all began in January of 1995. I was a computer scientist leading research projects for NASA. My husband Steve also worked in the computer industry, as a researcher for Apple Computer. I had done my doctorate work at Stanford University in the late 1970s and early 1980s, and since that time, both Steve and I had been active participants in the whirlwind of technology and innovation that is Silicon Valley. As we labored away in our cloistered research labs, friends and acquaintances were busy starting companies destined to become household names.

I also just happened to be a fairly knowledgeable devotee of modern medicine. An avid "Dr. Mom," I slept with a medical reference, the *Merck Manual,* on my night table. As I pored over this tome in the wee hours of the night, Steve would often ask, "Amy, why don't you just go to medical school?!"

Our two young sons, Izaak and Max, were six and three years old at the time. Naturally, we took their health needs very seriously. We would never hesitate to go to doctors when a problem arose, and we would invariably follow their advice without question. Unfortunately, we were also in the midst of a medical crisis. Our younger son Max was inexplicably afflicted with autism. This tragic and supposedly incurable disorder dramatically limits a child's ability to communicate and connect with others. And for some reason, it is mysteriously striking more and more children each year. Given the limited options for treatment, we were coping as best as we could.

By January of 1999, only four years later, everything had changed. I was now the mother of two sons progressing nicely through grade school. Max was no longer autistic — he was bright, talkative, and sociable. His autism had been cured with a controversial medicine of the past — *homeopathy*.

There were other changes as well. After two decades of research work, I had left computer science completely. I was now a student, editor, writer, and promoter of homeopathic medicine. The rest of my family was healthier than they had been in years. We used homeopathy as our primary form of medicine and viewed conventional medicine as appropriate only in life-threatening or time-critical emergency situations. I would no longer dream of doing things I had done routinely for years — suppressing fevers with aspirin or acetaminophen, coughs with cough suppressant, skin problems with cortisone, or combating ear infections with antibiotics.

What happened?

This book will reveal to you my own journey of discovery and healing, as well as that of my family and many friends. My goal is to share with you some surprising and truly revolutionary information that I have learned about the medical philosophy and healing power of homeopathy. In general, I have found that most Americans know very little about this form of alternative medicine. Though many people have heard the term "homeopathy," most confuse it with the use of herbs or think it is some kind of catchall term for natural or holistic medicine.

Of course, homeopathy *is* holistic (i.e., it understands and treats disease as a whole-body phenomenon), and homeopathic remedies *are* derived from natural sources. But it cannot simply be equated with these concepts. Homeopathy is a very distinct and complete system of medicine based on a simple principle of healing called the *Law of Similars*. This law states that *a disease can be cured by a substance if that substance can cause, in a healthy person, symptoms similar to those of the disease*. In fact, that is what the word "homeopathy" literally means — similar (homeo) suffering (pathy). While other holistic health-care systems are based on different principles or on accumulated experience and folklore, homeopathy, by definition, is the system of medicine based on this one cardinal principle.

As a medical discipline, homeopathy is certainly much better known and better accepted in other countries than it is in America today. It is widely practiced in Europe, India, Pakistan, and Latin America. In France, it is estimated that 32 percent of family physicians use homeopathy [Bouchayer]; in England, 42 percent of physicians refer patients to homeopaths [Wharton]. Homeopathy is integrated into the national health-care systems of many countries, including Germany, India, Brazil, Mexico, Pakistan, Sri Lanka, and the United Kingdom. Indeed, homeopathy is one of the four most widespread approaches to medical treatment in the world, alongside traditional Chinese medicine, herbal medicine, and conventional medicine [Poitevin].

Homeopathy is also a proven medical system. Hundreds of double-blind, placebo-controlled studies have been conducted over the past few decades, especially in Europe and India. They have proven that homeopathic remedies are indeed effective medicine. Wayne Jonas, MD, former director of the Office of Alternative Medicine at the National Institutes of Health, is one of the American medical researchers actively studying homeopathy. He has coauthored a book about homeopathic research studies [Jonas&Jacobs] and was also a member of a research team that analyzed 89 double-blind studies of homeopathic treatment; they found that homeopathy was, on average, more than twice as effective as placebo

[Linde]. Jonas's work, as well as several other research studies, will be discussed at length in Chapter 7 of this book. That chapter also takes a deeper look at just how homeopathic remedies might work. For now, though, let's take a closer look at what homeopathy is all about.

HOMEOPATHY'S PROMINENCE IN 19TH-CENTURY AMERICA

Ironically, homeopathy was quite familiar to Americans of the 19th century. In the late 1800s, there were more than 20 homeopathic medical schools in the United States. Homeopathy stood alongside *allopathic* (conventional) medicine and *eclectic* medicine (similar to today's herbalism or naturopathy) as one of the three accredited and accepted branches of medicine in this country. In fact, America was the world's leader in homeopathy at the time.

Where did homeopathy come from? Unlike many other alternative therapies that have become popular in America today, homeopathy is a Western medical system. It was developed by European physicians of the early 1800s who were discouraged with the results of the accepted medical practices of their time. A whole community of these homeopaths made their way to the United States in the 1830s and built strong practices and medical societies. In fact, the very first medical association of any kind in the United States was a homeopathic medical association — the American Institute of Homeopathy, founded in 1844.

Many of America's homeopathic medical schools still exist today, though all were converted to allopathy (conventional medicine) in the early 1900s. For example, the highly respected Hahnemann Medical School in Philadelphia was named for the founder of homeopathy, Samuel Hahnemann, MD. The study of homeopathy was still required at this school up until 1940, and homeopathic electives were taught until 1955. Other existing medical schools that began as homeopathic medical colleges include New York Medical College, the Boston University School of Medicine, and the medical school at the University of Michigan, Ann Arbor [Winston].

The very first woman's medical college in the United States was also homeopathic — the New England Female Medical College, founded in 1848. Homeopathy was the favored medicine among educated women of that period, and most of the early women physicians in this country were homeopaths. Even suffragist and feminist philosopher Elizabeth Cady Stanton was a talented lay homeopath. She was probably introduced to homeopathy by her brother-in-law, Edward Bayard, MD, a prominent homeopathic physician. Stanton's famous colleague, Susan B. Anthony, was also a proponent of homeopathy, her personal physician being homeopath Julia Holmes Smith, MD, of Chicago.

It is amazing that a medicine that was such an intrinsic part of 19th-century America became nearly forgotten in the 20th. Pioneers carried homeopathic medical kits as they traveled across the continent. Indeed, homeopathic remedies were often the only effective medicine available to them. The first American domestic manual (a medical reference for use in the home) was a homeopathic reference — *The Domestic Physician*, published in 1835 and written by Constantine Hering, MD, the father of American homeopathy.

Several American presidents, politicians, and the social elite of the late 1800s and early 1900s also used homeopathy. It was particularly favored by members of the new Republican party that swept into Washington in the 1860s. To this day, a statue of Hahnemann stands in Washington, D.C. — one of the only monuments in that city dedicated to a nonmilitary or nonpolitical figure. The statue was erected in 1900 at the intersection of 16th Street and Massachusetts Avenue, and its site was selected personally by President McKinley so that it could be seen from the White House. An avid supporter of homeopathy, McKinley was also the guest of honor at the monument's opening ceremony [*Homeopathy Today*].

In the early 1900s, homeopathy was still sanctioned and powerful enough to merit official status within the armed forces. For example, during World War I, there was a homeopathic medical corps — U.S. Army Base Hospital No. 48 — staffed by 100 nurses, 22 physicians, and two dentists, nearly all homeopaths [Bautista]. In 1922, President Harding, whose father served as a homeopathic physician in the Civil War, hosted a convention of homeopaths at the White House.

Homeopathy's popularity in the United States grew rapidly during the 1800s despite vigorous political and social opposition from allopathic physicians. This was largely because of its superior results. In the late 19th and early 20th century, homeopathic physicians and hospitals were known to have greater success in treating epidemics than their allopathic counterparts — for instance, in the 1832 cholera epidemic. In the deadly flu epidemic of 1918, the "Great White Plague" that claimed over 500,000 lives in America alone, homeopaths had a death rate of only 1.05 percent, whereas, overall, allopaths had a death rate of 30 percent — with reports of 60 percent not uncommon [Perko]. The charity hospital on Wards Island in New York City had the lowest percentage of deaths in that city. It was overseen by health commissioner (and later U.S. senator) Royal Copeland, MD, who used homeopathy for all cases [Winston].

Unfortunately, for reasons political, financial, and social, homeopathy was attacked and suppressed in the United States. The American Medical Association (AMA) was formed by the allopaths in 1847, partially in response to the threat of homeopathy. Its charter implicitly forbade members to associate either socially or collaboratively with homeopaths. Throughout the mid and late 1800s, the bans on contact with homeopaths escalated, and several allopaths were expelled from medical societies upon failure to comply. In his excellent book on the history of homeopathy in the United States, Julian Winston writes:

> "By the mid 1850s all state medical societies except the Massachusetts Medical Society had purged their homeopathic members. In 1856, the American Medical Association resolved that homeopathic works should henceforth no longer be discussed or reviewed in allopathic periodicals. After this time there was no formal communication whatever between the two branches of the profession; allopaths were forbidden to consult with homeopathic physicians or to patronize their pharmacies... In 1878 a physician was expelled from a local medical society in Connecticut for consulting with a homeopath—his wife... One of the leaders in Washington was Tullio Verdi, the first homeopath appointed

to the bureau of health in Washington, D.C., and the physician to Secretary of State, William F. Seward. When Lincoln was assassinated, there was also an attempt on the life of Seward. The White House doctor attended Seward, and informed Verdi, when he arrived, of what he had done. For 'consulting with a homeopath,' the White House doctor was severely censured by the Washington Medical Society." [Winston, pp. 51, 57]

Homeopathy was a threat to allopaths not only because of its therapeutic successes, but also because homeopathy's ranks were filled with MDs who had abandoned allopathy for homeopathy. They were rebels from within the fold. In contrast, eclectic physicians were primarily lay (non-MD) practitioners who posed less of a threat to the allopathic establishment. This legacy of acrimony between homeopaths and allopaths is forgotten by the American public today. But the history remains.

By 1950, there were barely 100 physicians practicing homeopathy in the United States, and they were, for the most part, old and close to retirement. The reasons for this decline are multifaceted and still debated among homeopathic historians to this day. Most agree that there were several contributing factors.

• The introduction of new allopathic medicines and techniques (aspirin, antibiotics, and the use of X rays and vaccination) made allopathy much more successful than it had previously been. Allopathy was also easier to practice and much more financially lucrative. Because homeopathy requires individualized treatment for each patient, it tends to be time-consuming. There are very few circumstances in which a homeopath can say, "Just take this medicine for that condition." Instead, remedy selection is tailored to the unique symptomatic profile of each patient. This makes homeopathy a much more arduous medical art, as well as much less financially profitable than allopathy.

• Social and political pressures on homeopaths to stop practicing homeopathy were enormous, fed financially by the growing power of the AMA and the allopathic drug manufacturers.

- There was infighting among the homeopaths themselves. Much of this was fueled by the increasing tendency of some homeopaths to use the new allopathic medicines, which supplied a much easier and quicker "fix," even if they did not cause as profound and long-lasting cures. As a result, a growing rift appeared between the classical "pure" homeopaths and the "half" homeopaths. Over time, allopathic-homeopaths also began to use homeopathic remedies in ways that were not in accord with classical homeopathic philosophy.

- Educational opportunities for the proper training of new and competent homeopaths declined precipitously due to decreased funding and school closures. Much of this occurred after the release of the Flexner Report in 1910. Commissioned by Andrew Carnegie in cooperation with the American Medical Association, the goal of the report was to rate or assess America's medical schools. Because the chosen standards were biased in favor of allopathy, the homeopathic schools were destined to lose out. Harris Coulter, PhD, a leading historian and writer about the politics of American medicine, and an expert on the homeopathic/allopathic rift, writes:

  "The findings of the Flexner Report, and the ongoing evaluation of medical schools by the American Medical Association, were soon accepted by state examining boards which decided to bar the examination to graduates of schools receiving a low rating — regardless of the candidate's own knowledge or proficiency. The refusal of examining boards to admit the graduates of schools which the AMA held in disfavor was the death-knell for these schools, and in this way the AMA acquired a whip hand over the whole medical education system, not only allopathic, but homoeopathic and Eclectic as well, a power which it had been seeking for decades." [Coulter73, p. 446]

In essence, the results of the Flexner Report barred those who attended homeopathic medical schools from obtaining medical licensure at all. But it wasn't only the Flexner Report that caused the demise of the homeopathic medical schools. The truth is, after the turn of the 20th century, less and less "pure" or classical homeopathy was taught even at these homeopathic institutions. Although there were still quite a few classical practitioners in the early 1900s, the majority of homeopathy's ranks had become allopathic-homeopaths. As a result, their therapeutic results began to suffer. Over time, the classical homeopaths died off and homeopathy became coopted by allopathy.

HOMEOPATHY RETURNS

Today, in a world dominated by a medical establishment that is increasingly technological and yet also increasingly unsatisfying, homeopathy is finally making a comeback. In the early 1970s, several young American doctors, most of them from the San Francisco Bay Area, were frustrated with the inability of allopathy to cure chronic disease. In the afterglow of the Sixties, they rediscovered the forgotten texts of the 19th-century homeopaths — and their discovery was revelatory. They saw in the old medical art the potential for a new way.

These aspiring new homeopaths quickly realized that there was no time to waste; they sought out the few remaining homeopaths in the United States and studied with them. They also made their way to Europe to study with teachers there, where homeopathy had remained a small but flourishing community. Indeed, it was the royal families — particularly the British royal family — that still championed homeopathy. Several of these young doctors also traveled to India, where homeopathy had become a popular medicine for the masses. Largely due to their efforts, as well as a growing interest in homeopathy among other kinds of alternative practitioners, a renaissance in American homeopathy began to emerge.

Today's small but growing group of American homeopaths is a varied bunch. There are licensed MDs, acupuncturists, osteopaths, and chiropractors who have begun to use a bit of homeopathy in their practices after some limited training. Some of these practitioners have delved deeper and now practice exclusively as homeopaths. Another group of practitioners are naturopaths — eclectic practitioners trained in a variety of healing modalities including homeopathy. Finally, there are professional homeopaths. These practitioners train specifically as homeopaths and are certified and represented by organizations such as the Council for Homeopathic Certification (CHC) and the North American Society of Homeopaths (NASH).

Unfortunately, there are also many individuals who market themselves as "homeopaths" but possess no homeopathic education or credential and, in fact, utilize techniques that have nothing to do with homeopathy. One reason for this is that homeopathic certification standards are not yet legally recognized by any state. In fact, there are still very few states where *anyone*, even a licensed medical practitioner, can practice homeopathy legitimately. Indeed, there have been MDs who have been charged with "unprofessional conduct" for practicing homeopathy, since it represents a "departure or failure to conform to the standards of accepted and prevailing medical practice" [Winston, p. 440].

Given this situation, it isn't surprising that there aren't many homeopaths practicing in America; there are currently fewer than 400 certified professional homeopaths in all of the United States and Canada. Despite the public's steadily increasing use of alternative medicine [Kessler] and the popularity of homeopathic remedies in health food stores, the serious professional practice of homeopathy in the United States is still very much in its infancy. Indeed, homeopathy's ranks are much smaller than those of other unlicensed alternative therapies. Why? One reason may be the extensive education and effort required for effective homeopathic practice. Another reason may be more political and cultural: lingering acrimony from the allopathic-homeopathic rift of the past.

HOMEOPATHY — THE "BLACK SHEEP" MEDICINE

Homeopathy's "black sheep" status among alternative therapies became clear to me one evening in 1996, when I attended a conference on consciousness studies in Tucson, Arizona. I had ended up in the company of a group of allopathic physicians who were deeply interested in psychic phenomena. Over dinner they discussed amazing things they had witnessed or heard about — healings by shamans, distance healing with prayer, and more. I felt certain that these allopaths would at least be open-minded about homeopathy. When I proceeded to tell them about the miraculous cure of my son and about my intention to begin studies in homeopathy, they stared at me blankly. "Oh Amy. Don't study *that*! Study Chinese herbalism or acupuncture instead." Their reaction startled me. These doctors could accept the potential validity of "psychic surgeons" from the Philippines, but they could not even consider a form of medicine that had been practiced with success for two hundred years, largely by MDs, in Europe and America. But perhaps that was why they could not consider it. It wasn't exotic enough. It wasn't Oriental or shamanistic. It was a Western alternative that had sprung up in their own backyard — a rebel from within.

Actually, there are many reasons why today's allopaths tend to be skeptical about homeopathy. On a superficial level, allopaths claim that homeopathy cannot possibly work because there is no known explanation for its mechanism. Most homeopathic remedies are made from mineral, plant, or animal substances that have been diluted using a process called *potentization*. Because these remedies are so dilute (they contain, from a biochemical standpoint, not even a single molecule of original substance), most doctors and scientists cannot see how they can be anything but ordinary water. But recent studies (which will be discussed in Chapter 7) show this not to be the case — something about the water in these ultradilutions *has* been discernibly altered.

Of course, the skeptics are also partially right — it is most likely that homeopathic remedies do not operate biochemically and according to any known mechanism. Their action is probably like that of other forms of *energy medicine* — for instance, acupuncture, which also does not operate biochemically or mechanically (despite the use of needles); Qigong, a Chinese meditative system that improves body energy flow; and hands-on healing methods like Reiki.

Requiring the mechanism of homeopathy to be scientifically explained before it can be deemed acceptable is also a bit hypocritical. Very few of today's alternative therapies have a known or accepted mechanism of action. The mechanism of action of many allopathic medicines is not understood either. Indeed, if every scientist believed that something *could* work only if they knew, a priori, *how* it worked, most scientific discoveries would never have been made. Did we know how electricity worked before we harnessed and used it? Do we deny that gravity "works," even though we still don't know exactly *how* it works? As Aristotle wrote in his *Nicomachean Ethics* (I.vii.17–18):

> "Nor again must we in all matters alike demand an explanation of the reason why things are what they are; in some cases it is enough if the fact that they are so is satisfactorily established."

Invariably, when skeptics find that homeopathic remedies do actually cure, they resort to the next most popular argument against homeopathy — that its effectiveness is due to the "placebo effect." In other words, they claim that the remedies are irrelevant; the patient has healed themselves by "the power of suggestion." Tell that to the victims of the 1918 flu epidemic! Obviously, the placebo effect of homeopathy was far more effective than the "real" medicines and suggestions of allopathic doctors. And tell that to the many sufferers from chronic illness who have recovered completely under homeopathic treatment, when the best that allopathy could offer was years of increasingly ineffectual symptomatic relief.

Why would the placebo effect work for homeopaths when the suggestions of allopaths hadn't? How does the placebo effect work on herds of cows that are cured of mastitis when homeopathic remedies are put into their drinking water [Spranger]? How does it cure newborn infants? Indeed, why do homeopaths often have to try several remedies before they find one that actually cures? If it was all "suggestion," wouldn't the first remedy work, regardless of what it was?

Of course, the so-called placebo effect is, in fact, a powerful healing force — the ability of the body to heal itself. And it is used by all healers, including allopaths. From this standpoint, the skeptics are probably right. Homeopathic treatment most likely does operate by harnessing the body's innate ability to heal itself. But a recent research study that collectively assessed a group of homeopathic clinical trials found that, overall, homeopathic remedies were *more than twice as effective as simple placebo* — a rate of success that would be enviable in many conventional allopathic drug trials [Linde]. And, increasingly, more successful studies are being done by medical researchers each year.

Naturally, the bottom line is that most of today's allopaths don't know very much about homeopathy. This was certainly true of the doctors I had dinner with in Tucson. But even if they were better educated, most allopaths would have difficulty accepting homeopathy — because its basic tenets and philosophy are at odds with everything they have been taught.

For one thing, homeopathy is not "complementary" to allopathy. It can't merely be viewed as a helpful adjunct to conventional treatment, like massage or chiropractic can be. Rather, homeopathy is a complete and *alternative* system — one that is able to treat the full range of physical and mental afflictions, from ear infections to allergies, from asthma to tuberculosis to psychosis. Although the two systems of medicine can often be made to work together at a practical level, homeopathy and allopathy are intrinsically incompatible at an ideological level. This makes homeopathy difficult for many people, and especially allopaths, to accept.

For instance, if homeopathic doctrine is correct, two of the primary tools of allopathy — *suppressive medications* (which remove the symptoms of disease, even if they cannot actually cure it) and *routine use of vaccinations* — are destroying our collective health in slow and insidious ways. According to homeopathic philosophy, suppression or repeated palliation (i.e., temporary removal of symptoms) can lead to deeper, more intractable forms of disease. For example, it may be this year's use of cortisone cream for eczema that eventually leads to the development of asthma next year. Homeopaths also believe that the routine and blanket use of vaccines, without a threat of imminent infection to balance their effects and without attention to the individual characteristics of each patient, can lead to damaging and lasting ill effects on health. What allopathic doctor wants to believe this? And yet there are a growing number of young American physicians, trained in the best of modern allopathic medicine, who have abandoned their training and embraced homeopathy, just as their counterparts did in the 1800s.

Ask yourself. As a society, are we healthier than we were 50 years ago? Today, a majority of Americans suffer from some form of chronic condition — a condition that, according to modern medicine, can only be palliated or suppressed, not cured. The *Journal of the American Medical Association* reported in 2002 that 80 percent of adults in the United States now take some form of medication each week, with 50 percent taking a prescription drug [KaufmanD]. Rates of chronic childhood disease have skyrocketed; asthma, attention deficit disorder, autism (once incredibly rare), learning disabilities, chronic ear and respiratory infections, severe allergies, and diabetes have become commonplace. Among adults we have an increasing number of cases of lupus, multiple sclerosis, chronic fatigue, depression, fibromyalgia, and chemical sensitivities.

What is going on? Could it be that our societal tendency to take a pill to suppress every cold and cough, an antibiotic to stamp out every infection (whether necessary or not), a cream to suppress every eruption, and a vaccine to combat every disease (whether or not the disease is typically benign or the person is actually at risk), has created this situation? The scary answer may be *yes*. And let's not forget the increasing levels of toxins, antibiotics, and hormonal agents in our food and environment. Even farm animals are subjected to vigorous suppressive drugging regimes.

Unfortunately, the increased trust and reliance of the public on modern medicine has led us into a reckless willingness to ingest scores of pills without a second thought. We even buy weekly pill organizers to keep it all straight. Why? Many of us find reassurance in scientific tests of efficacy. But the truth is, the therapeutic effects deemed acceptable for many drugs are often quite weak — only two or three percent improvement over placebo in some cases. Moreover, the assessment of side effects for most treatments is usually quite short-lived — just a matter of days or weeks. What are the real consequences down the line? Can we even measure them?   Even more frightening, it has been increasingly acknowledged that many drug studies are biased because the researchers who perform them are financed by the manufacturing drug companies.

Sadly, we find all too often that yesteryear's "scientifically tested" and much heralded treatment is now considered to be horribly dangerous. It stands to reason then, that treatments considered essential and safe today may be considered extraneous or dangerous next year. Indeed, the pace of this turnover seems to have accelerated with the increasing number of drugs that are turned out by the pharmaceutical industry. It seems that nearly every week some previously touted "wonder drug" later emerges as a threat to public health. A study published by the *Journal of the American Medical Association* in 2002 predicted that nearly 20 percent of new prescription drugs will ultimately be recalled or will be shown to produce unacceptably harmful side effects [Lasser]. Even the most standard treatments for ailments like asthma can change radically in a short period of time. Will Taylor, MD, an American allopath-turned-homeopath, wrote in 1998:

> "The half-life of conventional medical knowledge, and consequently of any standard of care, is approximately three years and growing short-er. It is rather amusing to me to watch the trends of therapy proposed by a discipline that, at any point, insists so vociferously on its omnis-cience. Back in my residency (in the 1970s), in treating asthmatic crises, we used to pay so much attention to theophylline levels and intravenous theophylline drip rates — a medicine that recent con-trolled clinical trials tell us is not effective in the treatment of asthma. That doesn't help me feel too confident in the therapies that have been proposed to replace it." [WT1]

Of course, allopathy can be a lifesaver when it is truly needed in an emergency. And some form of vaccination or prophylaxis may be appropriate in some circumstances. But our increased willingness and desire to pop a pill to suppress all symptoms, stamp out all germs, and artificially build up our antibodies with vaccines may be making us all sicker. And what about the new and more virulent diseases emerging each year — diseases for which there are no vaccines or treatment?

The real solution to our ever-increasing health problems might actually be found if we redirect our focus: from the "bugs" and stress outside ourselves, to our own ability to cope with them. *How can we strengthen ourselves?*

It is interesting that the philosophical tenets of homeopathy, known in the 1800s, would have easily predicted our current situation: an increased use of suppressive medicines ultimately leads to an increase in chronic disease. Luckily, homeopathy also provides a solution. The route to cure is the appropriate use of a remedy that is *homeopathic* to a sufferer's symptoms. This remedy can strengthen and enable an individual to heal. It can also provide a patient with a greater ability to meet the physical and emotional challenges that occur each day. Ironically, homeopathy, the "black sheep" medicine of the 1800s, may actually be one of the only means available to us for strengthening ourselves so that we can survive the challenges of the new millennium.

What You Will Find in This Book

To date, most popular books about homeopathy have focused on the curative powers of specific homeopathic remedies or on the treatment of specific ailments. In contrast, the primary goal of this book is to introduce you to homeopathy's way of thinking about health, disease, and cure. You will also read many amazing cure stories — the homeopathic experiences of my own family, as well as the experiences of many other people, suffering from a variety of ailments. This book will also provide guidance to you if you decide to seek homeopathic care for yourself. You will learn what to expect and how you can best benefit from homeopathic treatment.

Structurally, I have tried to organize the book as a journey of discovery. You will learn about homeopathy in a way that parallels the path of development of homeopathy itself — following in the footsteps of Samuel Hahnemann as he discovered and developed the tools and concepts of the homeopathic system. Let's begin with a short summary of what's in store for you. (Or, feel free to turn right away to Chapter 2.)

Chapter 2 begins with the story of Samuel Hahnemann, MD, the founder of the homeopathic system. It includes colorful details about his life and the times in which he lived, and provides insight into the tenacious and brilliant nature of his mind — a mind that never stopped searching for a true path to cure.

Ultimately, it was Hahnemann's tenacity that led him to discover the central tenet of homeopathy, the Law of Similars. As mentioned before, this law states that *if a substance can cause the symptoms of an illness in a healthy person, it can cure those symptoms in a sick person.* For example, suppose that a particular substance, X, is given experimentally to a set of healthy test subjects. During this test, X is found to temporarily cause symptoms of asthma such as tightness in the chest and difficulty breathing. It is also found to cause other physical, mental, and emotional symptoms — for example, certain kinds of digestive problems, headaches in a particular location and at particular times of the day, and a feeling of depression each day after lunch. Now, suppose that we have an actual asthma sufferer, Ms. Jones. If Ms. Jones experiences the same kinds of physical and emotional symptoms that X caused, then X has the potential to cure her asthma as well as her other matching symptoms.

The Law of Similars essentially defines what homeopathy is. The word "homeopathy" (sometimes spelled "homoeopathy") literally translates to "similar suffering." In the example above, substance X is *homeopathic* (i.e., causes a similar state of suffering) to the disease state of Ms. Jones. Therefore, X has the potential to cure (i.e., remove) this state, not just control or palliate its symptoms. A homeopath, by definition, is a practitioner who treats people according to this principle.

After exploring the context in which the Law of Similars was discovered, **Chapter 3** brings you back to today's world and reveals to you my own family's homeopathic experiences. The story of my son's amazing

cure from autism is fully described, along with anecdotes about the healing of other friends and family members. These healing stories, along with
others provided throughout the book (and especially in Chapter 9), illustrate the philosophy and principles of homeopathy in practice.

Chapter 4 then asks you to take a step back and consider some fundamental questions. What is health? How and why does disease develop?
What are the signs of true cure? Homeopathy views the body and mind
as an integrated dynamic unit rather than as a set of individual plumbing parts. This body/mind unit is seen as a physical and energetic system
that acts as a whole, responds to stimuli, and changes over time. By carefully observing how patient health tends to evolve over time, homeopaths have been able to gain a deep understanding of how disease
develops and how it recedes. As a result, they are more able to accurately assess a particular patient's present state of health, as well as the success
or failure of treatment.

For example, suppose that a patient's gastrointestinal problems seem
to have been cured by some treatment. How do we know if this person
has been truly cured and is becoming healthier, or is actually getting
sicker in the long run? Rather than viewing the patient's gastrointestinal
problems in isolation, a homeopath will watch to see what symptoms
arise next. What if the patient next develops a deep depression that was
never experienced before? Or, alternatively, he or she begins to manifest
skin problems that had occurred two years ago? These two outcomes
would mean completely different things to a homeopath. The development of depression would be a sign of deepening disease and therefore
unsuccessful treatment of the gastrointestinal problems. The return of old
skin problems would be a sign of return to greater health. The reasons
why this is so is the subject matter of homeopathic philosophy — the
primary topic of this chapter.

Next, **Chapter 5** focuses on the singular nature of disease. Not only
is each person a dynamic, holistic entity, but he or she is unique. Because
of this, each patient will express their sickness in their own way —
through the lens of their personality, their habits, and their unique state

of being. This is easy to see on an emotional level. Everyone knows that when a person falls sick, they will tend to react in a way that is individual to them. Some people withdraw, some beg for consolation, some become fearful, some go into denial. Everyone is different. Individualization occurs on a physical level as well. For instance, some people feel better when lying down and wrapped up in blankets. Others are relieved by moving about or from a nice cool breeze.

Of course, most people have unique peculiarities, even when they are well. For example, they may have food cravings and aversions, a preferred sleep position, or a particular pattern of sweating. Some people dress warmly, even on a hot summer day. Others run around in shorts in the middle of winter. Each person has a unique psychological approach to life as well, influenced by their experiences and the adaptations they have made to survive those experiences.

It is specifically this unique physical/mental/emotional gestalt that a homeopath is looking for when they try to find a matching remedy for a patient. Although the typical symptoms of a patient's diagnosed disease are taken into consideration, these symptoms carry less weight in making a homeopathic prescription than they do in making an allopathic prescription. For example, a homeopath who treats a hyperactive child will not be so interested in the fact that the child runs around a lot and has trouble staying focused. That is how most hyperactive children behave. Instead, the homeopath will try to understand this child's individual expression of hyperactivity. What situations make her worse or better? What are her peculiar mannerisms, fears, likes, and dislikes? It is these symptoms that form the basis for a homeopathic prescription. There may be 50 remedies that can be helpful for hyperactivity. Which remedy will cure a particular child will depend on his or her unique traits and habits. Because of this, homeopathy is a very individualized form of medical treatment. Each person, no matter what their diagnosed disease, will receive a remedy that matches them as an individual.

How did Hahnemann develop homeopathy as a complete system of therapeutics? **Chapter 6** takes us back once again to the early 1800s, the time in which Hahnemann and his growing group of followers expanded the homeopathic system. The chapter begins by describing how the ultradilutions of homeopathy were discovered and how Hahnemann developed principles for administering them. These include the use of the *single remedy* (only one remedy at a time) and the use of the *minimum dose* (the smallest amount necessary). Chapter 6 also briefly describes various schools of homeopathy that have developed over time and how they differ from one another.

Next comes **Chapter 7**, a chapter that will be of particular interest to the skeptical or scientifically minded reader. It begins with a description of several scientific studies that support homeopathy's efficacy. It then addresses the question: *how does homeopathy work?* The current answer is, we don't really know. But recent research studies seem to indicate that electromagnetic effects may be involved, and that the structure of water in homeopathic ultradilutions may actually carry a characteristic electromagnetic signature. If this is true, it doesn't matter if there is no molecule of original substance left in a remedy; some form of signature of that original substance may be present.

Even though the action of homeopathic remedies remains unexplained, most homeopaths have developed a variety of models or ways of understanding how they operate. Most of these models rely upon a construct called the *vital force* or *dynamis*— a concept analogous to Chinese medicine's *qi* or Indian medicine's *prana*. The vital force is considered to be an energy that animates each living creature and is the place where physical, mental, and emotional problems originate. Thus, a physical symptom — for example, a tumor — is viewed as the end result of a disturbance in the vital force, not as the root cause of disease in itself.

It is also in this dynamic realm that the remedies are considered to operate. Somehow, they are able to restore an adaptability that the vital force has lost, and enable it to function normally once again. Unlike traditional Indian or Chinese medicine, however, homeopathy does not structure the vital force into any kind of "energy anatomy" consisting of chakras or meridians. Nor does a specific model of the vital force form the basis for treatment — as it does, for example, in acupuncture. Rather, the only basis for the selection of a homeopathic remedy is the Law of Similars. Thus, homeopathy is a system of energy medicine based purely on the observed empirical effects of remedies on the human body and mind.

At this point, you will have come to understand much more about the history and philosophy of homeopathy. **Chapter 8** will then describe the experience of homeopathy — what it's like to be a homeopathic patient. A person coming to a homeopath for the first time will be surprised to find that this experience is much more like seeing a psychologist than a physician. An initial appointment typically takes one or two hours. During that time the homeopath will try to elicit as much information as possible about the patient's psychological and physical states and how they evolved over time. The goal, of course, is to understand the patient's symptoms deeply and completely enough to enable the selection of a remedy that is homeopathic or similar to them.

Because of this, a good homeopathic patient is one who facilitates the process by conveying as much information about themselves as they can — habits, fears, eating habits, sleep position — you name it. Indeed, information that would seem irrelevant to an allopath — a peculiar fear of dogs, a nail-biting habit, or the exact hour that symptoms tend to occur — can be critical to the selection of a homeopathic remedy. In fact, the more unusual or striking a symptom is, the more likely it will lead to the *simillimum* — the precisely matching remedy for a patient.

Chapter 8 also covers the line where allopathy and homeopathy inevitably meet. Some patients cannot be taken off their allopathic medications. And sometimes allopathic treatment is completely appropriate and necessary, even from a homeopathic point of view. Luckily, homeopaths are almost always able to work with patients under these circumstances, in collaboration with the treating allopath.

This chapter will also provide you with guidance in navigating through the homeopathic healing process. Many people come to a homeopath with chronic problems, after years and years of unsuccessful allopathic treatment. Ironically, such patients often expect to be cured quickly and easily, overnight. It is important to remain realistic. A disease state that has developed over several years will occasionally yield quickly to homeopathic remedies, but usually not. The process of homeopathic cure often has many ups and downs. For all of these reasons, homeopathic patients need patience, confidence, and sufficient education about homeopathy to determine if their case is truly progressing and is being handled appropriately.

This brings us to **Chapter 9**, chock-full of amazing cure stories. While the entire book is sprinkled with anecdotes of homeopathic cures, this chapter provides several additional stories that will hopefully convince you further that homeopathy is a complete and effective system of medicine.

So where does homeopathy stand today, and where should it be going? This is the focus of **Chapter 10**. Among the many challenges facing the American homeopathic community are the low numbers of well-trained classical homeopaths and the lack of educational facilities for training homeopaths in a complete and proper fashion. On top of this, little or no insurance coverage is available for homeopathic treatment, and there are very few states in which the practice of homeopathy, as a discipline in its own right, is truly legal. All of these problems must be addressed if homeopathy is to grow and flourish in this country, alongside the many other alternative therapies increasingly being used by Americans today.

The consumers of health care in the United States and around the world deserve the right to control how their bodies are treated and which form of medicine they choose. It is time for the powerful medical monopolies to be broken. In the 19th century, homeopathy, an inherently energetic system of healing, was perhaps before its time. Now that the philosophical ramifications of modern physics and quantum reality are beginning to enter our collective consciousness, it may finally be time for homeopathy to take its rightful place as a leading energy-based medicine of the 21st century. Indeed, homeopathy may be one of the only truly effective means we have for overcoming chronic disease and restoring our mental, emotional, and physical health. Shouldn't we have it available to us?

As Hahnemann said, *"Aude Sapere"*— Dare to know! So, read on and find out more about the fascinating and revolutionary world of homeopathy and how it could bring dramatic healing into your own life.

CHAPTER 2

)⸙

THE LAW OF SIMILARS

"The physician's highest and only calling is
to make the sick healthy, to cure, as it is called."

— SAMUEL HAHNEMANN, MD
First Aphorism, *Organon of the Medical Art,* 1810 [Hahnemann]

THE CREATOR OF THE HOMEOPATHIC SYSTEM, CHRISTIAN
Frederich Samuel Hahnemann, was born on April 10, 1755, in
Meissen, Germany. The Hahnemanns' family trade, the painting of porce-
lain, was severely disrupted by wars in that region and time. As a result,
young Samuel had to be educated mostly at home. Nevertheless, his
exceptional abilities soon became widely known. He had an extraordinary ability for independent study and critical thought. Rima Handley,
a biographer of both Hahnemann and his second wife, Melanie, writes:

"Days of studying on his own at home, and even at school, for he was
always far in advance of the other students, provided him with the
inclination as well as the capacity for independent thought, a trait
which was both to torment and sustain him in the years to come."
[Handley, p. 51]

When Hahnemann was 20 he embarked on his medical studies at the
university in Leipzig, which was considered to have the best medical faculty at the time. He made his living by tutoring German and French to
wealthy foreign students and by translating scientific texts. An adept student of languages (he was fluent in German, English, French, Italian, Latin,

and Greek, and was also knowledgeable enough to translate Hebrew, Chaldaic, and Arabic), scientific and medical translation became Hahnemann's stopgap means of earning a living for many years. Ultimately, one of the texts he translated would lead him to his discovery of the fundamental principle of homeopathy, the Law of Similars.

From the start, Hahnemann found the medical practices of his time to be questionable. Medical theories of that period focused on the balance of "humours" (fluids) in the body. Clinical techniques were primarily based on the idea that health could be restored by removing supposedly noxious fluids from the body. Thus, the most popular treatments tried to encourage sweating, vomiting, diarrhea, bleeding via cutting of veins (venesection) or the application of leeches, or the creation of blisters to draw inflammation from one part of the body to another. Sedation via opiates was also popular, as was the use of toxic doses of mercury in the treatment of venereal diseases.

One positive aspect of Hahnemann's medical studies was the influence of his teacher Hermann Boerhaave of Leyden. Boerhaave "maintained that the most important thing for a physician to do was to sit at the bedside of his patient and observe him in the manner recommended by Hippocrates." [Handley, p.52] This emphasis on an intense observation of the patient's symptoms became the foundation upon which Hahnemann based all his future work. It was his penchant for observation, coupled with a propensity for critical thought, that enabled Hahnemann, even at the start of his career, to see through the veneer of his time's accepted medical practices. He quickly realized that they were not only ineffectual, but even harmful.

By the time he was 29, Hahnemann decided that the best option for his patients was to simply let them heal on their own, rather than to administer the standard treatments. He became an outspoken proponent of natural healing techniques such as the adoption of a proper diet, the employment of good hygiene, and the improvement of poor living conditions — all common sense today, but not at the time. Pasteur's germ theory and antiseptic surgery were not to be discovered for another 80 years. Hahnemann soon gained a reputation as a dietician and wrote publicly about the importance of hygiene. This technique of cure came to be called "Hahnemann's Method" — long before his discovery of homeopathy. Hahnemann also became a proponent of the humane treatment of the insane, who were handled with utter brutality in that period.

By 1790, at the age of 35, Hahnemann had grown so disgusted with the methods of medical practice of his time that he completely gave up practicing medicine altogether. Instead, he turned to translation and his skills as a chemist to make a living. He wrote:

> "My sense of duty would not easily allow me to treat the unknown pathological state of my suffering brethren with these unknown medicines... The thought of becoming in this way a murderer or a malefactor towards the life of my fellow human beings was most terrible to me, so terrible and disturbing that I wholly gave up my practice in the first years of my married life... and occupied myself solely with chemistry and writing." [Haehl, p. 64]

As I will describe later, it was also in 1790 that Hahnemann got his first inkling about the Law of Similars.

Hahnemann the Rabble-Rouser

As the years passed and Hahnemann began to develop his own ideas about medical treatment, he spoke out more and more vehemently against the established medical profession. For example, in 1792, when Emperor Leopold II of Austria was bled to death by his doctors, Hahnemann wrote publicly about his views and caused quite a stir in the process.

> "We ask, from a scientific point of view, according to what principles has anyone the right to order a second venesection when the first has failed to bring relief? As for a third, Heaven help us! But to draw blood a fourth time when the three previous attempts failed to alleviate? To abstract the fluid of life four times in twenty-four hours from a man who has lost flesh from mental overwork combined with a long continued diarrhoea, without procuring any relief for him! Science pales before this!" [Haehl, p. 35]

Americans may be surprised to find out that their first president, George Washington, was also the victim of the same questionable but accepted medical practice of the late 18th century. In fact, Washington suffered the same fate as his counterpart in Austria.

On December 14, 1799, President Washington fell ill with a severely sore throat. One physician after another was called in to tend to him. Over the course of that day and after much discussion and argument, they agreed to drain the president of at least four pints of blood. To add insult to injury, they also gave him doses of calomel (a mercury compound used as a laxative) and tartar (to promote vomiting), and applied blistering agents to his legs and feet. Not surprisingly, this 'heroic treatment' — the common term used for this kind of medical care — led to Washington's death that night [Kaufman].

Of course, it seems obvious to us today that bloodletting isn't such a great idea. But at the time, any recovery that just happened to follow this procedure was attributed to the success of the method. When it failed and the patient died, a doctor could at least claim that he had done "all that he could." In truth, the same might be said of some of today's accepted medical practices. How often do we find that it is really the medical treatment that kills a patient rather than his or her disease? Is doing nothing the better option in some cases?

A chilling statistic reported in the *Journal of the American Medical Association* (JAMA) in 2000 provides support to this possibility; at least 225,000 deaths occur annually in the United States from the negative effects of medical drugs (106,000 deaths), hospital errors (27,000 deaths), hospital infections (80,000 deaths), or unnecessary surgery (12,000 deaths). This makes allopathic treatment the third leading cause of death in America [Starfield]. Only two years earlier, in 1998, another study reported in JAMA found that allopathic drugs were the fourth leading cause of death [Lazarou]. While most people trust that today's medical treatments have been proven safe and effective, the fact is, this is often not the case. Indeed, a 1978 report, "Assessing the Efficacy and Safety of Medical Technologies," compiled by the Congressional Office of Technology Assessment, found that only 10 percent to 20 percent of the techniques used by allopathic physicians are empirically proven [OTA].

Thus we can see that the struggle to find safe and effective medical treatments continues to this day. While the medical context in which Hahnemann lived may have been even more extreme and harmful than the one in which we find ourselves in today, the impetus that propelled him to find a better way, a more gentle and effective method of true healing, bears similarity to the quest of many people today for medical alternatives. And being of brilliant mind and stubborn temperament, he persevered in this quest, regardless of the consequences.

Another striking parallel between Hahnemann's time and our own is the enormous power of the orthodox medical establishment and especially the drug manufacturers. Just as it is today, medicine was big business in Hahnemann's time. Naysayers to the orthodoxy were not very popular, and they were often ridiculed and run out of town. Hahnemann suffered this fate for much of his life, especially after he began to practice homeopathy. He moved his family from town to town at least 18 times between 1782 and 1821. His most vociferous opponents were usually the apothecaries (pharmacies), not the doctors themselves. This was because Hahnemann prepared his own medicines. As a result, his popularity posed a threat to their business.

The same phenomenon can be seen today, with the financial stakes being even higher. Alternatives to expensive and toxic allopathic drugs, such as those used for cancer or AIDS, are routinely belittled and suppressed. In some cases, their proponents, even respected scientists and doctors, are threatened with legal prosecution and imprisonment. Two examples of this phenomenon are discussed at length in a fascinating article by medical historian Harris Coulter, PhD. One is the case of world-renowned physician and professor Andrew Ivy, MD, who was persecuted in the 1950s for his use of Krebiozen as an immunologically-based (rather than chemotherapy-based) cancer treatment. Another more recent case involved the harassment of Stanislaw Burzynski, MD, PhD, for his development of antineoplastons as a cancer treatment [Coulter98].

Sadly, throughout medical history, political and financial motivations have often outweighed therapeutic ones. Hahnemann was all too acutely aware of this phenomenon. Given the societal pressures to which he was increasingly subjected and the hardships his family suffered as a result, it was remarkable that Hahnemann maintained his views and continued to forge his own path.

DISCOVERY OF THE LAW OF SIMILARS

Once Hahnemann gave up practicing medicine, he soon became well known for his translation of a number of important medical and scientific texts. His translations were unique and sought after because he often added his own opinions and suggestions as footnotes. Throughout this period he also kept searching for a better method of healing — a system of medicine that made sense to him and worked in practice.

Luckily, fate was soon to catch up with Hahnemann when he translated the *Treatise on Materia Medica*, by William Cullen, a professor of medicine at the University of Edinburgh. Cullen described the use of Peruvian bark for malaria. This bark, also called *cinchona* or *china*, was a wonder drug of the 18th century. It is the source of quinine, a primary treatment for malaria to this day. Cullen's explanation for the successful action of cinchona was that it had a tonic effect on the stomach. But this did not make sense to Hahnemann. An avid student of Hippocrates, whose dietary, hygienic, and observational recommendations he had taken so seriously, Hahnemann was also aware of Hippocrates' statement that cure could be achieved in one of two ways: through the action of "opposites" (i.e., using a medicine that creates the opposite effect of the patient's symptoms) or through the action of "similars" (using a medicine that creates the same symptoms experienced by the patient).

Armed with Hippocrates' hypothesis, Hahnemann decided to put cinchona to the test. He systematically took overdoses of the drug and noted the results. He described these as follows:

"I took, for several days, as an experiment, four drams of good china twice daily. My feet and finger tips etc., at first became cold; I became languid and drowsy; then my heart began to palpitate; an intolerable anxiety and trembling (but without rigor [fever]); prostration in all the limbs; then pulsation in the head, redness of the cheeks, thirst; briefly, all the symptoms usually associated with intermittent fever [malaria] appeared in succession, yet without the actual rigor. To sum up: all those symptoms which to me are typical of intermittent fever, as the stupefaction of the senses, a kind of rigidity of all joints, but above all, the numb, disagreeable sensation which seems to have its seat in the periosteum [a membrane that covers bones] over all the bones of the body — all made their appearance. This paroxysm lasted from two to three hours every time, and recurred when I repeated the dose and not otherwise. I discontinued the medicine and I was once more in good health." [Haehl, p. 37]

This experience supplied a flash of insight to Hahnemann. He saw in it the potential for a general principle of cure — a medicinal law that always applied and worked, rather than a theory about how the body functioned or about a particular drug. This principle would become known as the Law of Similars. It states that,

A substance that causes, in a healthy person, symptoms similar to those of a disease state, can cure a sick person in that disease state.

In Latin this principle is written *similia similibus curentur* (i.e., "let likes be cured by likes"). Thus, just as cinchona caused the symptoms of malaria in the healthy Dr. Hahnemann (*note*: it did not cause malaria itself), cinchona could also cure a person afflicted with malaria.

Of course, Hahnemann wasn't the first to use this principle; Hippocrates himself had suggested it. Paracelsus, a renowned medieval alchemist and doctor, was also known to have achieved cure through the use of similars. In Hahnemann's own time, the writings of Antoon de Haehn (another pupil of Boerhaave) and a Danish professor, Georg Stahl, also emphasized the utility of this principle. Hahnemann, however, unlike the others, decided to put the idea to a full test and explore its limits. It became his life's work and the central tenet of his method of healing, which he called *"homoeopathy"* (now typically shortened to *homeopathy*) — "similar suffering."

DRUG PROVINGS

Critical to the successful application of the Law of Similars was developing a method for testing potential drugs and determining the symptoms that they could cause — and by inference, the symptoms that they could also cure. Hahnemann called these tests *provings* (derived from the German word for test, *pruefung*), and his test subjects *provers*.

From his experience with cinchona as well as the many other provings he conducted later on (during his lifetime he was involved in 123 drug provings [Provings]), Hahnemann found that it was important that these tests be conducted on healthy humans, not on sick humans or animals. Note that this strategy is the opposite of the one used by allopathic medical tests, which are conducted *only* on sick people or animals. Hahnemann wrote,

> "If, in order to perform this investigation, medicines are only given to *sick* persons (even when only one simple and singly prescribed medicine is given) one sees little or nothing definite of their pure actions since the particular condition-alterations expected from the medicines are mingled with the symptoms of the present natural disease, and are therefore seldom distinctly perceptible.
>
> Therefore there is no other possible way to unerringly experience the peculiar actions of medicines upon the human condition — there is no single sure, more natural arrangement for this intent — than to administer each single medicine experimentally, in a moderate amount, to healthy persons in order to learn what alterations, symptoms, and signs of its impinging action each medicine particularly brings forth in the condition of body and soul, that is, what disease elements each medicine is able to and tends to arouse. As has been shown, all of a medicine's curative power lies in its power to alter the human condition; this is illuminated from observation of the human condition." [Hahnemann, Aphorisms 107 and 108]

Thus, as Hahnemann explains, there are several reasons for conducting provings on healthy humans. First, if the true action of a drug is to be determined, it must be tested on a clean slate. If a prover is healthy, it is relatively easy to see what deviations from their original state are caused by a drug. In contrast, if a sick person takes a drug, their symptoms may be cured, aggravated, or new symptoms may result. In essence, the effects of the drug become mixed with the person's initial state of disease and a clear picture of its precise action becomes difficult to determine.

The disadvantages of using animals for provings are also clear. For one thing, determining the precise mental and emotional symptoms caused by a drug becomes almost impossible when provers are animals. Animal provers are also unable to describe the precise nature, location, and sensation of their physical symptoms. As I will discuss later on, homeopaths have found that emotional, mental, and precisely described physical symptoms are the most critical pieces of information gathered in drug provings — because these symptoms enable the most effective selection of remedies for patients. Animal provers simply cannot provide this kind of information.

Another disadvantage of animal testing is that we cannot be completely sure that the effects of a drug on an animal will be exactly the same as they would be in a human. Since homeopathic treatment is based on symptom similarity, it is critical that provings be conducted on creatures who are as similar as possible to patient clientele — i.e., humans. Nevertheless, homeopathic veterinarians have been fairly successful in using human proving symptoms to select appropriate remedies for their animal patients. In fact, several astounding veterinary cures are described in Chapters 7 and 9.

Over time, Hahnemann continued to further develop his proving methodology and to conduct new provings. He also enlisted the help of his colleagues. In 1813, when Hahnemann was a lecturer at the University of Leipzig, his core of followers formed a Provers Union. All of the myriad symptoms gathered during these provings were compiled as books called *materia medica*. As a translator, Hahnemann also had access to much of the medical literature of his time, and in particular, to records of accidental poisonings. These provided yet another source of information about the symptoms caused by potential drug substances. Over time, the homeopathic materia medica also grew to include *clinical symptoms* — i.e., symptoms that had been repeatedly cured by remedies in clinical settings.

From Hahnemann's time until this day, new provings continue to be conducted each year. Remedies are tested on healthy human subjects (usually volunteer homeopaths) and observations are made over a period of several weeks. In keeping with modern scientific methodology, today's provings are almost always double-blinded — neither the test subjects nor the people collecting the proving data know the nature of the remedy substance. Modern provings also usually include a control group, which takes a placebo instead of the drug itself.

PHILOSOPHICAL CONSEQUENCES OF THE LAW OF SIMILARS

Because the practice of homeopathy is defined by an underlying law of therapeutics, its very nature as a medical system is fundamentally different from allopathic medicine. Think about it. The Law of Similars specifies, in a general purpose way, which medicines will cure which disease states. In particular, to cure any disease with symptoms x-y-z, a homeopath must simply find a remedy that causes x-y-z in a healthy person. Because a fairly well-matching remedy can usually be found among the existing set of about 1,000 remedies, *a new type of treatment need not be found for every new type of disease.*

Indeed, because it uses a fixed and general-purpose law of treatment, the same homeopathic method can be applied in *any* case of disease and that method of treatment *never changes over time.* Though the number of available homeopathic remedies has increased over the years as a result of new provings, the fundamental principle of homeopathic practice has remained the same — the Law of Similars. As a result, the medicines tested and used by Hahnemann in the early 1800s still work today for the same disease states. And even though new diseases may be discovered each year, new remedies need not necessarily be developed to combat them.

In contrast, no overarching law of therapeutics exists for allopathy. Treatment is based either on theories about how the body or a disease agent works (theories that are inevitably incomplete and change over time), or on medicinal knowledge that is developed in an ad hoc fashion, through folklore and experience — whatever seems to work. A good example of this is Viagra, a medicine developed for treating circulatory problems that also just happened to cause erections. As a result, Viagra is now marketed for impotence, despite the fact that it may cause dangerous circulatory side effects.

What are the consequences of the allopathic approach? First of all, a new therapy must often be developed for each new disease or condition that is discovered. Second, the approach tends to create a medical system with constantly changing conventions of practice. This is as true (or perhaps more true) today as it was in Hahnemann's time. Back then, bloodletting seemed to have the desired effect and was therefore considered a well-grounded practice. Today, we have a never-ending stream of new drugs, many of which were developed almost by accident and many of which will be declared useless or harmful in just a few years.

The grounding of homeopathy in the Law of Similars also has an impact on the need to conduct conventional drug trials for homeopathic remedies. Homeopathy is often criticized by allopaths for being insufficiently tested with respect to specific diseases. Aside from the fact that such tests are now increasingly being conducted and successfully so (see Chapter 7), from a philosophical standpoint, conventional drug trials for homeopathic remedies are actually unnecessary. Because allopathic drugs are not applied according to a specific principle and are often discovered in an ad hoc way, it is clearly necessary to test them to see if they actually work. In contrast, the testing of a potential homeopathic remedy on healthy humans (a proving) is not only the most accurate method of determining what it will be useful for, but it is also a completely sufficient method of testing; *provings are homeopathy's drug trials.* There is no need to test remedies on sick people, because the Law of Similars specifies exactly which ailments a remedy will effectively treat — those whose symptoms match those caused by the remedy. And the Law of Similars *has* been proven valid — time and time again, over the past two hundred years of homeopathic practice.

HAHNEMANN'S PERSONAL LIFE

After his experience with the malaria drug cinchona in 1790, Hahnemann spent the next several years conducting drug provings on himself and on interested colleagues. Hahnemann and his followers also began to test the efficacy of the Law of Similars on patients. In 1796, he published his first treatise on his new method, *Essay on a New Principle for Ascertaining the Curative Powers of Drugs, and Some Examinations of the Previous Principles.* Finally, in 1797, at the age of 42, Hahnemann officially resumed his practice of medicine as a homeopath.

Unfortunately, life for the Hahnemann family became even more difficult after Samuel resumed his practice. The region was torn by unending wars and his large family moved frequently, due to financial problems and, increasingly, friction with the local apothecaries. Despite these disruptions to his personal life, Hahnemann worked tirelessly to develop new remedies and methods for administering them. He also "wrote article after article attacking what he called 'old school' medicine and advocating the new homeopathy, and published them in widely-read medical journals." [Handley, p. 68] This period culminated in the publication of the first edition of his full treatise on homeopathy, the *Organon of the Medical Art*, in 1810. It did not go unnoticed.

> "By its very nature, the whole of Hahnemann's new system threatened the prevailing system of medicine. He was no longer willing to accommodate the 'old school'; ... there was no compromise. Medical treatment which is not homeopathic is dangerous, he says, not merely when it is abused and used carelessly, or to excess, but when it is used at all... According to Baron von Brunnow, a young law student who

later became a patient of Hahnemann's in Leipzig, 'The appearance of the Organon was the signal for the actual breaking out of the war against Hahnemann. If the physicians had, up to that time treated his writings with haughty disrespect, and had regarded them as too insignificant for notice, they now felt for the first time that a dangerous antagonist was making head against them…They directed a broadside from all the great cannons of criticism against the daring revolutionist.'" [Handley, pp. 72–74]

In 1811, Hahnemann moved his family into the eye of this storm — Leipzig — after gaining faculty status at the university there. Considered an eccentric troublemaker, he nevertheless built up a loyal following. His popularity increased even further after the typhoid fever epidemic in 1813.

"The efficacy of homeopathy became particularly apparent in 1813, after the terrible Battle of Leipzig between the Prussian forces and Napoleon's army, retreating from the fiasco of Moscow. After three days of fighting just outside the city, there were 80,000 dead and 80,000 wounded. The streets were choked with refugees, it rained incessantly, food supplies were short and the drinking water polluted. Of the one hundred and eighty victims whom Hahnemann was able to treat, only two died… Hahnemann's success, however, only increased the anger of the orthodox. His flourishing practice in Leipzig also aroused opposition." [Handley, p. 76–77]

Eventually, the allopaths of Leipzig had their way. Because he prepared his own medicines, Hahnemann was brought to court in 1820 and accused of encroaching upon the apothecaries' privileges there. Eventually he had to leave Leipzig, and finally, in 1821, settled his family in Koethen in eastern Germany. Hahnemann was now 66. And despite these setbacks, his fame continued to grow. Students and open-minded physicians came to study with him from all over Europe. Patients flocked to him from afar. Eventually, Hahnemann's system spread to all of the countries of the European continent as well as England, America, and even India.

The following account, also by Von Brunnow, provides a glimpse of what Hahnemann was like as a man. Although he was definitely opinionated, strong-willed, and self-disciplined, he was also compassionate, somewhat eccentric, very sociable, and beloved by all who knew him.

> "'A very peculiar mode of life prevailed in Hahnemann's house. The members of his family, the patients and students of the University, lived and moved only in one idea, and that idea was Homeopathy; and for this each strove in his own way'... Hahnemann was able to relax at home in this supportive company, usually in his favorite 'gaily-figured dressing-gown, the yellow stockings and the black velvet cap. The long pipe was seldom out of his hand, and this smoking was the only infraction he allowed himself to commit upon the severe rules of regimen. His drink was water, milk or white beer; his food of the most frugal sort... After the day had been spent in labour, Hahnemann was in the habit of recruiting himself from eight to ten o'clock, by conversation with his circle of trusty friends. All his friends and scholars had then access to him, and were made welcome to partake of his Leipsic white beer, and join him in a pipe of tobacco. In the middle of the whispering circle, the Aesculapius reclined in a comfortable armchair, wrapped in the household dress we have described, with a long Turkish pipe in his hand, and narrated, by turns, amusing and serious stories of his storm-tossed life, while the smoke from his pipe diffused its clouds around him.'" [Handley, p. 76]

Hahnemann's life took an interesting turn in his last years. His wife Johanna died in 1830, when Hahnemann was 75, and he settled into a somewhat reclusive life with two of his daughters. Even so, homeopathy's fame continued to spread, especially after it met with great success in treating the European cholera epidemic of 1831–1832. In 1834, a beautiful and wealthy Parisian poet and artist, Melanie d'Hervilly, appeared in Koethen. She had read Hahnemann's *Organon* and had traveled in men's clothing across Europe (a custom in vogue among women of the intelligentsia) to receive medical treatment by the doctor. They instantly fell in love, despite their age difference — Hahnemann being 79 at the time, and Melanie, 34. Within three days he had proposed to her, and within three months, they were married.

Much to the surprise and consternation of his followers, Hahnemann moved with Melanie to Paris. She quickly became one of his best students and one of the first lay practitioners of homeopathy — and one of the first women to practice medicine in Europe. With her help, Hahnemann built a thriving practice that served both the rich and illustrious (among them, Paganini and Balzac) and the Parisian poor, in a clinic that Melanie ran herself. During these Paris years Hahnemann also continued his experiments, and he developed new and improved methods for remedy dosing.

Thus it was in Paris that Hahnemann, perhaps for the first time in his life, felt happy and relaxed. Compared to the difficult life he had lived up until that point, in Paris he enjoyed luxury and the company of high society. And he was deeply in love. As he wrote to Melanie in January of 1843, just months before he died:

> "I have no need to repeat to you that I love you with all my heart as I have never loved anyone throughout the whole of my long life. You are superior to everyone I can imagine loving because both your soul and your moral sense correspond to my own feelings. We shall never be parted throughout all eternity." [Handley, p. 153]

Samuel Hahnemann died on July 2, 1843, with Melanie by his side. He was 88 and she was 43. Melanie never remarried. She continued to practice homeopathy, despite years of harassment by the medical establishment, until she died in 1878. She is buried next to Hahnemann in Père Lachaise cemetery in Paris.

HAHNEMANN THE SCIENTIST

At this point, I hope that I have conveyed to you at least some feeling for what Hahnemann was like as a man, as well as the core essence of his medical system, homeopathy. Hahnemann was a scientist in the truest sense of the word. He began with observations and a theory and then set out to verify it. Whatever the outcome, he left preconceptions behind and went with experimental fact. And, being of stubborn temperament, he stuck by his findings, despite the criticism of his peers.

Throughout his life, Hahnemann kept experimenting and refining his system. It is through these experiments that he came up with the ultradilute doses that homeopathy is known for today. Because many of the remedies he used were innately poisonous, Hahnemann tried to find dosages that could be both effective and gentle. Toward this end, he began to dilute them to a greater and greater extent. Eventually, in 1810, Hahnemann developed a method for creating effective doses that were so dilute that not even a molecule of the original substance would likely be present. This point is reached when the ratio of water to substance is in excess of Avogadro's number (approximately 10^{23}). Interestingly, Avogadro's first hypothesis about molecular weight was first made soon thereafter, in 1811 [Furtsch].

Hahnemann's method for creating ultradilute yet effective medicines is called *potentization*. It involves not only diluting a substance, but at each step of dilution, *succussing* or violently shaking the solution. Homeopaths have always believed that it is this process of potentization that enable remedies to touch and affect the energetic realm of the vital force — the place where disease is believed to arise and where true cure must take place. However, it is only in the past 20 years that physicists and medical researchers have confirmed that succussion may be the essential step necessary for transmitting the signature of a substance into an ultradilution [Benveniste88, Ennis]. This research will be discussed in Chapter 7.

In addition to developing the potentization process, Hahnemann also experimented with a variety of methods of remedy preparation and administration. For example, he tried various different dilution ratios, amounts of succussion, and administration methods — dry pills, liquid, and olfaction (sniffing). As a result of these experiments, Hahnemann was able to delineate a set of principles for safe and effective homeopathic treatment. These include the use of the *single remedy* (administering only one remedy at a time, not in mixtures), and the use of the least amount of remedy necessary to cure — the *minimum dose*. Hahnemann's experiments with potentization and other aspects of remedy creation and administration will be described in more detail in Chapter 6.

Hahnemann's relentless desire to improve his system also resulted in many improved editions of the *Organon*, still the most comprehensive text on the principles and practice of homeopathy to this day. The first edition of the *Organon* appeared in 1810; ensuing editions appeared in 1819, 1824, 1829 (the first to be translated into English), and 1833. Today's homeopaths use the Sixth Edition, which was completed in 1842 but was not published until 1921, long after Hahnemann's death.

HOMEOPATHY AS EMPIRICAL MEDICINE

In many ways, Hahnemann can be considered a "radical empiricist" — a term coined by the late psychologist and philosopher William James. This means that he allowed for all forms of scientific evidence and that he was led by this evidence rather than by preconceptions or accepted scientific doctrine. For instance, like James, Hahnemann was willing to utilize subjective information from patients and provers — not just information that could be gathered by an outside observer. Indeed, Hahnemann found subjectively experienced symptoms to be more important than measurable or observable ones. For example, he found it more useful to know that a person subjectively felt hot or cold (and the exact nature of that hot or cold feeling) than to know the person's precise temperature reading on a thermometer.

One reason for the importance of subjective symptoms in homeopathy is that treatment is determined by matching the subjective symptoms of patients to the subjective symptoms experienced by provers — i.e., subjective feelings and expressions are matched to subjective feelings and expressions. For example, let's suppose that two remedies, *A* and *B*, are known to be useful in cases of fever. However, in the proving of *A*, a feeling of dry heat was accompanied by thirst and anxiety. In contrast, the provers of *B* felt sweaty, thirstless, and apathetic. By taking into account these subjective proving symptoms and comparing them with the symptoms of a feverish patient, a homeopath can prescribe *A* or *B* as the situation warrants. As a result, treatment can do more than just temporarily palliate a fever — it can cure it.

The homeopathic emphasis on subjective experience also points to another fundamental difference between homeopathy and allopathy: homeopathic remedy selection is based on the idiosyncratic symptoms of a person's disease state, not on its physiological cause. In allopathy, treatment usually depends on making a causal diagnosis. Disease must be reduced to some measurable pathology or dysfunction before treatment can begin. In homeopathy, a physiological explanation for disease is only a small piece of the disease puzzle. In a case of stomach ulcer, for example, the real question is, how does this ulcer fit within the patient's larger pattern of disease — a pattern that incorporates a variety of mental and physical symptoms, and of which the ulcer is only a small part. It is this pattern that is treated by the homeopath, not the ulcer.

This brings us to one final observation. Given the fact that the homeopathic remedies are probably operating on some kind of quantum or energetic level, it is quite fitting that Hahnemann's methods were focused on symptoms rather than on causal explanations. If, as homeopaths believe, disease truly originates and is ultimately cured in the realm of an intangible vital force, then all we *can* do is observe its manifestations; we can never hope to completely know its true cause, because it lies at a level of reality we cannot perceive. In his treatise on the relationship between homeopathy and psychotherapy, *Psyche and Substance*, Jungian psychiatrist and homeopath Edward C. Whitmont, MD, wrote:

> "...in modern physics we have come to realize that phenomena cannot always be explained in terms of a cause and effect chain... they can be predicted in their arrangement only statistically; and a field is defined not as it 'is' this or that, but only indirectly — that is descriptively — through the patterns and forms of matter that manifest its influence...We [homeopaths] assay the expression of an energy field of the illness, unknown per se, but found and manifesting itself in the way it arranges the symptoms." [Whitmont, pp. 4–5]

In other words, at the quantum level, all we can do is observe patterns. We cannot explain why a quantum pattern exists — we can only observe it. The homeopathic approach to disease reflects this principle by focusing on a patient's symptom pattern rather than on trying to determine its cause. The Law of Similars then asserts that bringing together similar patterns — the disease pattern of the patient and the disease pattern of a similar drug — will cause the patient's disease pattern to be annihilated. As a result, it is not necessary to know what caused a disease in order to cure it. It is enough to know that bringing together similar patterns will do so.

We opened this chapter with the *Organon's* first aphorism. We now conclude with a portion of Hahnemann's footnote to that aphorism. It touches directly upon this very same subject: the goal of finding a cause for disease versus the goal of simply trying to cure it.

> "The physician's calling is not to concoct so-called systems from empty conceits and hypotheses... it is not to make countless attempts at explanation regarding disease appearances and their proximate cause... Of such learned fanaticism... we have had quite enough. It is high time for all those who call themselves physicians, once and for all, to stop deceiving suffering humanity with idle talk, and to begin now to *act*, that is to really help and to cure." [Hahnemann, Footnote to Aphorism 1]

CHAPTER 3

ℐ

TESTIMONY TO CURE

"In the hands of a true Master, homeopathy holds the answer for the vast majority of chronic disease sufferers... It may seem too good to be true, but humankind's centuries of searching for a non-toxic, truly curative medicine have finally come to completion in the homeopathic system."

— BILL GRAY, MD, Foreword to *Homeopathy: Medicine of the New Man,* 1979 [Vithoulkas79]

ONE OF MY FIRST TEACHERS OF HOMEOPATHY TOLD ME THAT A person's views about homeopathy's curative powers tend to be colored by their first experience with it. For some, it is a cure of intransigent warts that suddenly dry up and drop off. For others, a case of shingles, allergies, migraine, or chronic fatigue yields and fades away, when years of other kinds of treatment had no effect. Then there are the cases that truly defy explanation: expulsion of a tumor; a man awakening from a coma minutes after taking a remedy; the discharge of mercury in the menstrual blood of a dental hygienist, after years of accumulation in her system. All of these have occurred with the correct homeopathic prescription.

Whatever the miracle may be, great or small, when you experience the power of an accurately prescribed remedy, you are forever changed by it. You may come away thinking, "Homeopathy is sure great for skin problems," or "These remedies can cure ear infections and stomach flus so quickly!" But no matter what you think, you are changed by that first curative experience. If an infinitesimal dose of plant, mineral, or animal matter can have such profound effects — a dose that, according to current scientific understanding, contains nothing at all — then things can't be quite as they seem. And something definitely must be lacking in the mechanical view of the body that we have all been brought up with in the Western world.

Of course, most of us fall back into old ways of thinking. When the next flu crops up, we just take an over-the-counter flu medicine without thinking that there might be another way. Often we doubt that our cure was real at all. "Well, surely that problem must have been all in my mind." "Most likely it was that new vitamin I took." "Maybe the drug the doctors gave me a year ago finally worked?" Or maybe we come away thinking that homeopathy is only good for some things. "It seems to be good for ear infections, but surely it can't cure my asthma." "It seems to be good for emotional or mental problems, but I don't think it could cure a bacterial or viral infection." But the more you use homeopathic remedies, especially under the direction of an experienced and well-trained homeopath, the more expanded your view becomes. Each curative experience renews a sense of wonder and awe at the kinds of healing that are possible.

The power of homeopathy has repeatedly had its impact on every member of my family and on many of my friends. I have seen long-standing warts suddenly turn brown and drop off like scabs — this happened to both my husband and to my older son Izaak. I have also seen fairly severe tics and twitching stop overnight, a bout of cramping and diarrhea that had persisted for several days disappear in minutes, and my own summer allergies suddenly vanish, after years of growing increasingly more severe. I have seen an ear infection in my son Max, visible with an otoscope, subside within hours; his outer ear went from bright red to a normal color within minutes too. In another case, a six-week bout of bronchitis — that did not yield to several homeopathic remedies — stopped completely, overnight, when the correct remedy was given. I have seen sexual arousal heightened, panic and anxiety allayed, and closed personalities open up and become more connected, loving, and sympathetic.

Interestingly, when I tell acquaintances that I no longer have to take a daily antihistamine to get through the summer, they are often more impressed than when I tell them about my first and greatest homeopathic miracle. My younger son Max was cured of an "incurable" condition — autism. Today, years later, I sometimes have a hard time believing it myself. We were very lucky, you see. Our homeopath found Max's *simillimum* — his perfectly fitting remedy — on the first try. Within a week, his therapist, my husband, and I were witnessing noticeable changes in him. Whatever may be said about Max's case, it is certainly true that something remarkable happened to him in 1995. And this initial experience with homeopathy most definitely colored my views about the kinds of cures that are possible — nearly limitless — if the body and its vital force still have the power to be led back and restored to health.

THE WARNING SIGNS

It all began in the spring of 1994, when Max was 2½ years old. Something wasn't right. He wasn't talking. Although he had about 10, maybe 20, words in his vocabulary, most of the time he didn't seem to understand language at all. And it was getting worse. On some level, Max seemed to be slowly drifting away.

On the bright side, Max did know all the letters of the alphabet and his numbers 1 to 10. He could stack blocks with amazing dexterity and could build highly intricate and perfectly symmetric structures. He even knew his way around the computer — pointing and clicking, dragging the mouse, and opening games. Max also displayed some amazingly advanced analytical skills. For instance, he could play a "Concentration"-style game, matching pairs of overturned tiles in a four-by-five grid, better than we could. And he could definitely hear. He enjoyed television and danced rhythmically to music. Indeed, for the most part, Max was a happy, though distant, toddler at home. He usually had a smile on his face and liked to play with his older brother Izaak — a precocious and mature 5½ year old.

But when we all sat around talking and laughing in the evening and on weekends, Max would prefer to be off on his own. He'd watch TV, play a computer game, stack his blocks, and retreat into himself. He also wasn't as affectionate as Izaak. Although he didn't push us away, he never reached out for affection. For a long time I thought, "Oh, he's just late to speak. He's a more self-contained, more private person than Izaak." But it was more than that.

At school, problems began to emerge. I began to sense that the teachers at his preschool were concerned. They greeted Max each morning with a kind of hesitancy. Although he had started the school year exuberantly at age two, he had never fully settled in. Instead, he would rely on his beloved "baba" — a bottle of milk — for comfort. And though he enjoyed many of the toys in the classroom, Max never interacted with any of the other children. He was also unable to sit through story-time unless he was in a teacher's lap. He was antsy, as if there were a motor running inside him. It wasn't like classic hyperactivity — he didn't run about. He just wasn't paying attention. It was as if the story the teacher was reading were in a foreign language. Left to his own devices, Max would just wander away and play quietly with toys that interested him. He wasn't disruptive; he just wasn't really "there." When the children were outside playing, the teachers would find him in a classroom raptly staring at some animal in a cage or at a toy.

I knew that one of the teachers suspected autism. She told me that Max manifested self-stimulation activities — for example, spinning in a circle — and that he didn't have good eye contact when spoken to. But I didn't want to believe it. He did have some eye contact with us at home. He didn't really spin around at home either; he was generally happy and content.

But increasingly, there were noticeable oddities. One morning while driving to school, I asked him, "Do you know where we're going now?" No response. Max just stared into space. At night, when I'd try to read a story to him, he could not sit quietly. He would fidget and squirm all over the bed. He'd stand on his head, with his feet against the wall, or run his fingers up and down things — the table, the wall. I also noticed that he had the habit of poking his finger against people's chests or butting his head against them — not to hurt them, but as a kind of contact. Over a year later, I learned that these behaviors are all characteristic of autistic children.

What to do? I began to grasp at straws. Perhaps it was attention deficit disorder (ADD)? I read all the books. Perhaps it was the teachers? That they didn't "understand" him? But deep down, I knew Max had a serious problem. And it seemed to be getting worse. He was growing more distant, more disconnected. By the end of the school year, just before Max turned three, the preschool called us in for a conference and advised us to seek medical help. One teacher confided to us, "Max will never be able to attend the private school that Izaak goes to. He will always need special education."

And so our family embarked upon a quest. I knew that we would never rest easy as long as Max had a problem like this; I knew that all of our lives would be severely affected. I felt instinctively that Max's entire future hung in the balance and that I had to do everything in my power, leaving no stone unturned, until I found the key.

My resolve was also deepened by another factor. This was one of my worst nightmares coming true. For years my mother and I had been deeply affected by my brother's struggle with severe mental illness. This past propelled me even harder to find a solution to Max's problem. I felt a call to arms, and in retrospect, it served me and my family well. I knew that there was no running away or avoiding the issue — no room for resignation. I knew that problems like this don't just go away; they cannot be ignored. I'd explore every nuance of our family dynamic, every food we ate, and examine every aspect of Max's life with a fine-toothed comb, looking for clues. This outcome for my son just didn't seem right to me. I was a mother on a mission.

THE SEARCH — WITHOUT AND WITHIN

In the summer of 1994, when Max had just turned three, we began to take action. On the advice of a speech-therapist friend, my husband and

I decided not to take him to the local child-development clinic affiliated with Stanford University that had been recommended to us. Our friend told us that they'd just label Max and create a sense of hopelessness in us. Instead, we took him to a highly respected speech and language therapist who runs a clinic in Palo Alto, Donna Dagenais. Donna was (and still is) considered to be the best language therapist in our area, with vast experience in working with children with communication and language disorders. She didn't label Max — she merely assessed him and set to work. In addition to his private therapy sessions, she also placed him in group sessions with two other children — including one who had already been formally diagnosed with Pervasive Developmental Disorder (PDD), mild autism. Of the three, Max was the best-behaved but the least verbal, and certainly the most "spaced-out."

Next it was food. In my reading about ADD, I had run across the recommendations of the Feingold diet for improving children's behavioral problems [Feingold]. One of the most suspect problem-foods was cow's milk. That sure rang a bell! Max was addicted to it. He had formed a "lovie" attachment to his bottle. When he'd watch TV, when we were in a car or plane, at all times of the day, he'd request his "baba." Some days he'd drink nearly eight bottles — half a gallon of milk. Perhaps this attachment was subconsciously related to the fact that, as an infant, Max had surgery for pyloric stenosis, a condition that closes the valve that controls the flow of stomach contents into the intestine. The most common symptom is persistent, violent vomiting. Because of this condition, Max increasingly threw up all the breast milk he drank during the first month of his life. Perhaps, after a month of not getting enough milk, Max enjoyed his milk all the more now.

In any case, Max's craving for and large intake of milk was certainly suspect. We took him off cow's milk and cut his consumption to one cup of goat's milk per day. This step alone had a dramatic effect. Before it seemed like Max was behind a curtain, living in a different world. Now, the first veil lifted. He finally began to talk and build two- to three-word sentences. And he was clearly more present, more aware of his world. His behavior and language were still by no means normal, but it was a start. By the end of the summer, we also began to limit his intake of artificial food colorings, another recommendation of the Feingold diet.

Interestingly, a recent study has linked some cases of autism to a kind of brain-reaction to milk protein. This study will be discussed later on in this chapter, as well as the possibility that this reaction might be triggered by childhood vaccinations. Certainly, cutting down on Max's intake of milk did create a dramatic change in him. But it did not cure him.

In the fall of 1994, Max continued his speech and language therapy with Donna and, after testing, qualified for special education benefits. He made slow progress. Despite the fact that he could now talk, Max still had a decidedly autistic interaction style. For example, he could only answer questions of the most literal kind, and only about objects directly in front of him. Thus, he could answer the question, "What color is this block?" but he could not answer an abstract question like "What is your favorite color?" He also had another autistic symptom — *echolalia,* or speech echoing. Rather than answer a question, he would sometimes merely repeat the last few words the other person had said. For instance, if you said to him, "Say good-bye," he would reply, "Say good-bye." Sometimes this was a remarkably effective strategy for him: "Do you want to go outside or stay inside?" "Stay inside." But soon we realized that he was merely parroting our words. If we asked the same question in a different way, his answer would change: "Do you want to stay inside or go outside?" "Go outside."

During the fall of 1994, we intensified our examination of our family dynamic and other social factors in Max's life. On Donna's advice, we took him out of his play-oriented nursery school and enrolled him in a Montessori school. The Montessori framework is extremely structured and focuses on reading and mathematical and manipulatory skills — things that Max was interested in. It also encourages children to do their work completely on their own. This was perfect for Max, who could not interact well with other children but could work fine alone. The school did not see him as disabled but simply as quiet.

Next, we looked deeper at our family dynamic. At the time we were using a nanny for child care three days a week. Steve and I each worked four-day workweeks so that one of us could stay home with the children the other two days of the week. Our nanny was a somewhat-distant young woman with health problems of her own. Fortuitously, she left the area at just around this time, and we were able to find a new nanny who was extremely sweet and loving. We encouraged her to focus a bit more on Max than on his highly verbal and engaging brother. Indeed, this was one of the challenges confronting me and Steve as well. We realized that we had to make a concerted effort to spend more concentrated and focused time with Max. It was often easy to "forget" him — he was always wandering off to be by himself. So we decided to take turns, each spending intensive time with one child or the other.

Finally, and perhaps most importantly, we examined ourselves — our own feelings and attitudes toward Max. Deep down, I realized that I had feelings of rejection toward him in his current state. It can be truly difficult to be genuinely accepting and loving when dealing with this kind of situation. Yet children with challenging problems are the ones who need the most from us. They are also the ones who are most psychically sensitive to parental feelings and attitudes. I instinctively knew that I had to cultivate a state of unconditional acceptance and love toward Max, and that this acceptance was critical for his recovery. I also knew that I had to truly believe, to have true confidence, that he *would* recover. Steve helped me a great deal in this regard. Somehow, he always knew that things would turn out all right.

HOMEOPATHY

It was now January of 1995. Curled up in bed, I was reading the latest issue of *Mothering*, a progressive parenting magazine. It included an article by Judyth Reichenberg-Ullman, ND, about homeopathy for childhood behavioral problems [Reichenberg-Ullman95]. She claimed that she was able to create substantial improvement in ADD cases 70 percent of the time. Since then, Reichenberg-Ullman, along with her husband Robert Ullman, have published a series of successful books about homeopathic treatment, including *Ritalin-Free Kids* [Reichenberg-Ullman96] and a new book about the treatment of autism and Asperger's syndrome [Reichenberg-Ullman04].

Back then I knew nothing about homeopathy. Although I had read Deepak Chopra's books about alternative methods of healing [Chopra], knew a bit about ayurveda (traditional Indian medicine), and had taken classes in Qigong and Tai Chi Chuan (Chinese disciplines to improve the flow of body energies), I thought, like most people, that homeopathy was some kind of herbal medicine. Occasionally I had taken over-the-counter homeopathic remedies for colds, but I didn't really know anything about homeopathy.

As I read Reichenberg-Ullman's article that evening, I was filled with an increasing fascination and excitement. I'll never forget the moment I finished reading it. A bell went off in my head. I knew that something important had happened. Little did I know that our lives were about to change forever. "Read this!" I said to Steve. The next morning I called an acupuncturist friend of mine and asked her where I could find a homeopath. She referred me to John Melnychuk, a professional homeopath new to the Palo Alto area. We quickly got an appointment and went with high hopes and expectations.

John is now a close family friend. Many years later, he told me that he was a bit stumped the day Steve, Max, and I walked out of his office in January 1995. Max was surely in an autistic state, but what other symptoms did John have to work with, besides those that were simply common symptoms of autism?

You see, although the nature of a patient's chief complaint or disease can be helpful in selecting a remedy for them, the symptoms that are merely typical signs of the disease aren't always that useful. As I will discuss in Chapter 5, the most fruitful symptoms are those that are *peculiar* to the individual. For example, nearly anyone with asthma will have difficulty breathing coupled with some anxiety about their condition. What will be most useful to a homeopath in choosing a remedy, however, will be that which is *unusual* about the patient and their asthma. The more peculiar or characterizing of the patient, the more useful a symptom will be in guiding a homeopath toward a precisely individualized remedy. Symptoms as peculiar as *"asthma, during the full moon"* or *"asthma, worse when listening to music"* can be found in the homeopathic literature. Such symptoms are usually associated with only one or two remedies that could be truly curative to a patient who experiences them. In contrast, a shallow or "routine" prescription for asthma, based only on common asthma symptoms, will most likely only palliate asthmatic symptoms, much as allopathic medicines do. Only a remedy that truly matches the person as an individual will actually cure them.

Given Max's youth and withdrawn state, it was a bit difficult to find symptoms that were particularly unique to him. However, some of the things that stood out included: his strong craving for milk, coupled with the fact that it aggravated his condition; his love of dancing and music; the tendency for his head to become very sweaty when sleeping; his preferred sleep position (on his back with his hands over the top of his head); his restlessness and intensity; a family medical history of both cancer and diabetes on Steve's side of the family and schizophrenia on my side; and a stubborn, perfectionistic, yet sweet personality. For example, during that first interview, Max became upset when he didn't successfully write "Mom" on a piece of paper just the way he wanted to.

All of the above characteristics are associated with the remedy that Max ultimately was given — *Carcinosin*. It is a relatively unusual remedy, but it is not uncommonly used in such cases. Of course, other remedies have been used successfully in autism cases as well. The key is to find the remedy that best matches a child's unique symptomatic profile.

Ultimately, what clinched John's recommendation for Max was a particular symptom that he found in a homeopathic *repertory* — a reference book that provides a reverse index to the materia medica. This symptom was associated with only one remedy, and it read:

"Talented, very: Carcinosin."

Apparently, I had mentioned 10 times during the initial interview that Max was talented! Perhaps I was an overly proud mother, defensive of her "special-needs" child. But I was quite certain of his innate talents. His observational skills and memory for visual detail were (and still are) quite extraordinary. He could watch television and perfectly imitate nuances in various characters' behavior and mannerisms. He could memorize dance routines and perform them for us. Even today, Max has an extraordinary memory for visual detail. He can watch a fast-paced cartoon and remember, days later, every bit of action that occurred. At age eight, he saw an interesting geometric figure within a painting on the wall of a restaurant, and remembered this same figure as the logo of another restaurant we had eaten at only once before — a month earlier. In recent years, he has emerged as a talented artist, with a flair for comic drawings.

As it turns out, Max had many other symptoms that are characteristic of Carcinosin as well. Because this remedy turned out to be his simillimum, I went on to study it further and write journal papers about his case for the professional homeopathic community [Lansky]. Introduced as a remedy in the early 20th century, Carcinosin was relatively unknown until D. M. Foubister, MD, a British physician, began utilizing and writing about it in 1958 [Foubister]. Its many symptoms include ones that Max also exhibited: bluish sclera (i.e., the whites of the eyes have a bluish cast); a tendency to have numerous dark-brown macules (large freckles); a hairy back and legs and heavy eyebrows; a craving for salt, butter, and spicy foods; perfectionism and tidiness; oversensitivity to reprimand or criticism; and a love of animals. Even Max's "poking" behavior, so common among autistic children, is described in one article about Carcinosin that appeared in the July 1963 issue of the *British Homoeopathic Journal*:

> "I have noticed that Carcinosin often has bizarre tics; one of my patients constantly tapped his brothers' skulls with his fingertips; another used to gently bite the tips of children's fingers, one after the other." [Hoa]

Of course, my goal here is not to go over all of Max's and Carcinosin's symptoms. It is merely to illustrate the kinds of symptoms that play a role in homeopathic prescribing. It is not a formulaic "take this for that" medical system. That's what makes it so hard to practice well.

INITIAL CHANGES

Max began taking his remedy on a Thursday morning. John had recommended a liquid dosing regimen — a kind of slow-and-steady approach — where a small amount of remedy, diluted in water, is given on a regular basis. In Max's case, we gave him a teaspoon each morning. Each time we gave him a dose, we also tried to imbue it with our love and good intentions.

Two days later, Steve and I began to notice some changes. Max was using some phrases he had never used before and was somehow a bit more socially aware. It was subtle, but something had definitely shifted. We also noticed that his speech was slightly more fluid. Usually, he spoke in a kind of "cogwheel" fashion — as if he had to think about each word he said. Over time, we found that noticeable and sudden improvements in speech and social awareness became Max's earmark for the effects of the remedy upon him.

The following Tuesday, five days after starting the remedy, Max had a session with his therapist Donna. We did not tell her about the remedy, but she quickly noticed that something had changed. "What did you do?" she asked. One of Max's exercises was to try to follow a list of instructions, such as "Put the ball on the red chair and bring the green block to me." Usually he was able to follow only a single command, rarely two. Suddenly he was able to perform two commands consistently.

And the trend continued. Each day we saw just a bit more improvement. As time went by and we went through successively increased potencies of the remedy, we began to see a definite pattern of response. A bottle of the remedy usually took a month to finish. When we began a new bottle, containing a slightly higher potency of the remedy, Max would show some increased signs of hyperactivity. These aggravations were not extreme, but they were noticeable to me and Donna. This period would usually last three to five days. It was followed by a sudden jump in verbal, cognitive, and social ability — a discrete and noticeable step upward. At this point, the hyperactivity would also tone down. Max would become more contained and relaxed. This was followed by a period of gradual improvement for about two weeks. At the end of the month, as we neared the end of the bottle, we would begin to see a gradual slipping backward. Donna and I used to call this Max's "end-of-the-bottle" behavior. This heralded the need to move on to the next potency level.

Skepticism

After a few months, the changes in Max had become quite noticeable. However, being scientists, Steve and I were naturally a bit skeptical about the whole affair. Was it the remedy that was changing Max? Was it our own expectations and attitudes? We decided to conduct a simple and, admittedly, not totally rigorous test. For two weeks, I would make daily observations about Max and write them down. Steve would give Max his morning dose, changing from one potency level (bottle) to the next, at a time unknown to me. The bottle would be hidden. Truthfully, I expected Steve to change bottles fairly early on in the two-week period. Each day I made my observations and jotted them down, straining to see that sudden shift, but seeing none. However, on the second to last day of the experiment, it happened — I noticed a sudden improvement in Max's speech. And, indeed, Steve had changed bottles three days earlier.

As it turns out, our skepticism about the miracle happening before our eyes was not that unusual. Over the past few years, I have seen several striking homeopathic cures. In those cases where the true simillimum has been found, the curative process is usually so natural and graceful that it seems that the person is just "getting better" by themselves. Of course, this *is* what happens; a remedy enables the body to heal itself. It does not "do" something to the body in the way that allopathic medicines do. It does not force a chemical change, so the body will not feel forced. For this reason, a person who is accustomed to the action of allopathic medicines will often think that a remedy did nothing; they will feel that they just "got better." Or they might attribute their cure to something else. But in truth, an appropriately selected remedy in the appropriate dose *should* be so gentle and effective that the person feels they just got better.

Of course, there are also situations where an inappropriate remedy or an inappropriate dose is given. In these cases, a person will either feel that nothing has happened at all, or, if they are sensitive to the remedy, that something unpleasant has come over them. For example, my mother once experienced a week of recurring mild fevers that began an hour after ingesting a remedy given in too high a dose. On another occasion, I found myself sitting and crying over some cooked onions that had been thrown away by mistake. Puzzled by the way I was overreacting, I suddenly realized, "Of course! I took a high dose of *Ignatia* [a grief remedy] yesterday." There I was, conducting my own personal proving of Ignatia, grieving over lost onions.

Interestingly, people often do not attribute these negative effects to a remedy either — they just don't feel like allopathic-drug side effects. Luckily, such reactions usually disappear soon after a remedy is discontinued or after potency or dose is adjusted. However, such phenomena do underscore the importance of treatment under the guidance of a trained homeopath.

Because Max's cure seemed so natural and proceeded fairly gradually, it seemed to many of our friends and family that he just grew out of his autistic state. But those of us who saw him almost daily — Steve, Izaak, our nanny, our housekeeper, Donna, and I — saw the direct correspondence between changes in dose and improvements in behavior. Donna, who is extremely experienced with children like Max, repeatedly assured me that what happened to Max was atypical. When he was clearly better, after a year of daily dosing (at which point we discontinued the remedy altogether), she confided to me that Max had been autistic. She said that she had seen autistic kids improve before, but not lose their autism like Max did. In fact, our pediatrician made the same confession. Once Max was better, she admitted that he had been autistic. She was quite surprised by the change in him. Many years later, when I brought the boys in for a checkup, she commented that she was still amazed at what had happened to Max.

OSTEOPATHY, REIKI, AND PRAYER

Six months after starting on Carcinosin, Max continued to improve in his ability to speak and understand language. His social awareness improved as well. However, much of his inner restlessness and social distance remained. When he was four, about six months after starting homeopathic treatment, I took Max to see a traditional osteopath on John's recommendation. While most osteopaths in the United States (with the DO credential) function as allopaths, a traditional osteopath heals only through hands–on manipulatory techniques. One of the goals of treatment is to balance and free the flow of cerebrospinal fluid, through very gentle, sometimes almost imperceptible, manipulations of the cranium, spine, and sacrum.

Max had a course of three osteopathic treatments in a month, followed by an occasional treatment once every few months. After his first examination, the osteopath felt that Max had signs of cranial compression, which he was able to correct. And indeed, Max's initial response to treatment was striking. While the homeopathic remedy had its primary effect on his language production, comprehension, and social awareness, osteopathy created the first major shift in Max's desire for physical affection. It also seemed to create a calming effect in him, quelling that sense of internal restlessness.

The night after his first osteopathic treatment, Max crawled into my lap and said, "Mommy, sing me 'Rock-a-Bye Baby'!" Although he did not usually push me away, this was the first time he directly asked me for this kind of physical loving attention. From that point on, Max did. Soon he began crawling into bed with me in the morning and snuggling at bedtime. He also began to run after me or my husband when we left the house to make sure he got that extra kiss good-bye. What a change from the distant "self-contained" Max!

Throughout the healing process, I also prayed for Max on a regular basis. When times were particularly rough, I would go into his room while he was sleeping and use a form of therapeutic touch called Reiki [Stein]. I truly believe that the effects of prayer and hands-on healing are not to be underestimated. In fact, an increasing number of studies have proven the beneficial effects of both on cases ranging from open-heart surgery to AIDS [Targ]. Many nurses are training in the use of such techniques and are beginning to use them in hospital settings. In my own experience, osteopathy, hands-on energy work, and prayer all work marvelously with homeopathic treatment. They seem to be complementary, boosting each other's beneficial effects.

JOINING THE CROWD

In the fall of 1995, after nine months of homeopathic treatment, Max began his second year at the Montessori preschool. At this point, his speech had definitely become more complex, spontaneous, and fluid. Donna tested him again and found that he was approaching his age level. She decided to discontinue therapy but kept him "on the books" as far as eligibility for special education.

Now that Max was talking, he was also trying to join in with the other children socially. But he was behind. Having started so late, he was awkward in his initial attempts at social interaction. He was stubborn and cried too easily when he didn't get his way. To get attention and acceptance, he often resorted to excessive silly "toilet talk." Of course, as a parent, I was thrilled that he was beginning to reach out to other children. But the school was not as supportive. They had pegged Max as a quiet child and did not like the new changes they saw in him. They gave him no support in his awkward transition from social withdrawal to social acceptance and savvy. One of his teachers said to me, "Max was such a nice boy before. Can you put him back the way he was?"

Although it was difficult to change schools in the middle of the school year and cope with this teacher's attitude, I had learned by this point that not changing to meet Max's needs would stall his progress. It was clearly time for some changes on the school front. So, at age 4½, we found a new school for Max — a more socially oriented school that followed the Montessori style, but not as strictly. His new teachers had no preconceptions or biases toward him, and they easily helped Max adjust. Within a few months he knew everyone at school, was interested in what was going on around him, had a couple of friends, and was having play-dates.

During that school year we also made some more changes on the home front. When our nanny decided to leave her position to follow her dream to become a beautician, Steve and I decided to stop using nannies altogether, opting instead for after-school child care three days per week. This change had many beneficial side effects for our family. For one thing, we finally began to eat dinner together every night as a family. Given the hectic schedule of families with two working parents, the institution of the family meal has gone by the wayside in many American homes. Returning to it created a feeling of greater coherence and stability in our lives. It also assured a better diet for our kids.

REMEDY ADJUSTMENTS, AND A HINT OF VACCINATION DAMAGE

By the end of 1995, it became increasingly clear that Max was being aggravated more than helped by his remedy. He was consistently more hyper and revved up. We began to decrease the frequency of his dose, but the aggravation remained. Finally, in January 1996, a year after Max began homeopathic treatment, we stopped it completely.

Sure enough, just like Max's marked improvement with each monthly change of dose, going off the remedy now led to a huge leap in language and social ability. This leap continued for about four months until it evened out. Max calmed down and his true personality began to emerge full force. He is an entertainer. He is sociable and sensitive.

Although he was still immature at this point, he was ahead of his peers academically. He was respected and liked by both his teachers and class-mates. In May 1996, Donna tested Max once more. He was testing above his age level! On the day that Steve and I joyfully signed papers releasing Max from eligibility for special education, Donna told the county social services representative that it was not her therapy that had done the trick for him; it was homeopathy. She also invited John and me to present Max's case to her clinic, which we did that summer.

Max was now almost five years old, and it was tempting for Steve and me to believe that he was fully cured. However, John was less sure, and he turned out to be right. There were still vestigial signs of his for-mer autism, though they were not readily apparent. For example, his lan-guage production continued to be awkward at times. In times of stress (for instance, if he was sick), he would retreat into himself and use echolalia as a speech strategy.

But overall, Max was functioning extremely well. He engaged in real discussions with family and friends. He asked for explanations about his body and his environment. He related stories about his day at school and about TV shows. He was also fascinated with fantasy play and dress up. Max was even becoming popular at school, with children running up to him and greeting him. He was able to adjust easily to new social situa-tions in the summer of 1996, readily adapting to two new summer camps. Max had also become an avid reader — another Carcinosin qual-ity. Before he began kindergarten he could already read simple Dr. Seuss books.

However, by the end of the summer of 1996, I began to notice a slight decline in Max's speech and social awareness. It also happened to be time for his five-year-old checkup at the pediatrician. And for the first time, I declined the routine vaccinations. At age five, it is customary to give the full battery — measles, mumps, rubella (MMR); diphtheria, pertussis, tetanus (DPT); and polio. Having read about a possible link between autism and vaccination damage, I didn't want to rock the boat. Our pediatrician did not argue with my decision either. But she did convince me to give Max the tuberculosis (TB) test that is required for kindergarten entry in California — now administered as an injection rather than the old tine test.

Unfortunately, this injection led to a marked aggravation and deterioration in Max's state. For the next week, he became increasingly sensitive, crying for no reason. The teachers at his camp and at school remarked about the change in him. He had become more withdrawn and fearful. He was not his new usual self. This reaction made us wonder if, indeed, vaccination was the root cause of Max's problems in the first place. Years later, I discovered another hint of this. After going through his medical records, I realized that at age 18 months, Max had been given a dose of the MMR (measles, mumps, rubella) vaccine only one week after recovering from roseola — an ailment related to measles. Perhaps he had been in a compromised state. Indeed, the MMR vaccine has been highly implicated in triggering autism [Wakefield].

Luckily, after a couple of tries with other remedies, our homeopath suggested that we simply return to Carcinosin. After a single dose, Max was back to normal within hours. We breathed a sigh of relief. Max started back on the remedy and remained on it for another eight months, once again changing potency level about once a month. Again we saw the same characteristic monthly pattern of response. After eight months, in March of 1997, I readily recognized the consistent aggravation and stopped the remedy. And once again, this was followed by a long period of noticeable improvement.

AN ONGOING PROCESS

Since that time, Max has no longer needed daily doses of Carcinosin. Just like the rest of our family, he visits our homeopath and osteopath about two times a year, or when the need arises. Sometimes he receives a remedy to deal with minor behavioral or emotional problems that crop up. Sometimes he receives a remedy when he gets an infection or virus and needs a bit of extra help getting over it. The same is true for me, Steve,

and our other son Izaak. We are all part of an ongoing process of healing and growth.

In the fall of 1997, I felt that Max was ready to leave his Montessori
school. At age six, he entered first grade at the private school that Izaak
attended. Since then he has done well both academically and socially. He
is an open-hearted, sensitive, and somewhat-comedic fellow who loves
drawing and art (he is especially fond of the quirky and enigmatic paint-
ings of M. C. Escher), playing computer games, reading fantasy and sci-
ence-fiction books, and writing and illustrating his own works of
science-fantasy.

But like all children, Max is growing and changing and occasionally
needs homeopathic and social supports. When he was in second grade,
input from his teachers alerted us to the fact that he was still having
some difficulty processing auditory input. For example, he sometimes
missed parts of oral instructions or key points in stories, especially when
they were read out loud to the class. Being quite sensitive to disapproval,
Max tended to cover up for these deficits and did not ask for help or
clarification from the teacher. The result was sometimes an excellently
executed assignment or essay, but written about the wrong topic. The
teachers were puzzled. Max's behavioral effect was normal, and his exe-
cution of assignments was always excellent if he understood what was
expected from him. There seemed to be something askew to them.

You see, up to that point, I had not told Max's teachers about his former autism. I didn't want to bias them in any way. And perhaps I wanted to forget about these problems myself. When these new issues arose,
I told the teachers about Max's history. As a result, they tried to provide
visual or written instructions for him when necessary, and occasionally
would check up on him to make sure he had understood class assignments. The net effect was excellent.

Max is now doing extremely well in life. After third grade, his audi-
tory-processing problems seemed to disappear, thanks to ongoing homeopathic treatment. His teachers no longer report any problems at all.
Today his behavior, demeanor, and day-to-day interactions with friends

and family are not in any way autistic. He's a sociable fellow with many friends and an excellent student working at his age and grade level. He takes piano and tennis lessons. He attends summer camps, including a monthlong sleep-away camp. He is resilient within his peer group, always able to defend himself with a kind of entertaining humor and charm. He is also a gentle soul, loved by his teachers. Of course, he still has his issues, like any other child. But we continue to work on them, and Max continues to improve. Invariably, his spirit and talents outshine any limitations. Max is no longer autistic, but he is still a "talented, very" child.

WHY AUTISM?

According to the Autism Society of America, between 500,000 and 1,500,000 Americans now have some form of autism. And the number is rising. Check around your community — autism cases are popping up everywhere. Every day I hear about more cases of this once incredibly rare and heartbreaking condition. In a statement to Congress in 1999 supported by the Central Missouri District School Nurse Association, Patti White, RN, estimated that the rate of autism-related disorders had risen in her district from 1 in 10,000 to 1 in 150 [White]. A 1999 California government report also found an alarming increase in the number of autism cases in that state. Two California state senators, John Burton and Wesley Chesbro, issued statements to this effect:

> "'In the past 10 years, California has had a 273% increase in the number of children with autism who enter the developmental services system — 1,685 new cases last year alone,' Burton said. 'What is generally considered a rare condition is increasing faster here than other developmental disabilities. We need to find out why.' 'The number of children with autism greatly exceeds the numbers you'd expect from traditional incident rates,' Chesbro said." [CalHealth]

In fact, in 2001, the U.S. Department of Health reported that the incidence of autism is rising at a rate of more than 20 percent a year [Herald].

Where did this alarming trend come from? As mentioned earlier, one proposed physiological explanation is a wayward reaction to milk protein. Two studies conducted at the University of Florida [Sun1, Sun2] have found that some autistic and schizophrenic individuals may lack the ability to break down proteins found in milk, possibly due to a malfunctioning enzyme. Research by a team that includes Dr. J. Robert Cade, the inventor of the Gatorade sports drink, found that:

> "When not broken down, the milk protein produces exorphins, morphine-like compounds that are then taken up by areas of the brain known to be involved in autism and schizophrenia, where they cause cells to dysfunction... Preliminary findings ... showed 95 percent of 81 autistic and schizophrenic children studied had 100 times the normal levels of the milk protein in their blood and urine... When these children were put on a milk-free diet, at least eight out of 10 no longer had symptoms of autism or schizophrenia." [Ross]

Now obviously, the recent dramatic rise in autism cannot simply be attributed to milk — something that children have always been consuming. What has changed is these children's ability to assimilate milk. Indeed, autistic children are known to be sensitive to many other foods as well — for example, wheat, gluten, corn, and food colorings — and their autism sometimes improves when these foods are eliminated from their diet.

But why have these food intolerances developed? One very compelling theory is that the ever-increasing use of vaccinations is to blame. Indeed, several studies and books have directly correlated the rise in autism — indeed, the very phenomenon of autism itself — with the introduction of the American vaccine program. The earliest reported cases of autism in the United States were in 1943, among affluent families — the families who were the first to give their children all the benefits of modern medicine, including vaccinations [Coulter90].

Since then, the situation has only gotten worse. It is now an incontrovertible fact that the incidence of autism, ADD, and other learning and behavioral disorders has risen precipitously over the past twenty years, along with a sharp increase in severe allergies and various other kinds of autoimmune disorders. This rise has occurred at the same time as the increased and mandated use of vaccinations for just about every childhood illness. Indeed, the number of different disease antigens (vaccine constituents that trigger an immune response) that are recommended for children by the time they are five years old has more than tripled in the last two decades [Mercola].

Can this correlation between an increase in vaccination and an increase in behavioral and autoimmune disorders be explained scientifically? Some scientists are starting to believe the phenomenon can be explained by the fact that vaccines stimulate a different branch of the immune system (the humoral or Th2 function) than is stimulated by actually experiencing a disease (the cell-mediated or Th1 function). As a result, it may be overstimulation of the body's Th2 function (by an ever-increasing number of vaccines) that may be causing wayward autoimmune responses [Incao]. Another popular theory is that various vaccine ingredients — mercury, in particular — are to blame. Some have also suggested a synergistic explanation — that toxins used in vaccines (such as mercury) increase the chance that wayward autoimmune reactions to immunization will occur [Haley].

Whatever the explanation, people are beginning to take notice. Missouri nurse Patti White's statement to Congress asserts her suspicions about the now-popular Hepatitis B vaccine. Once a staunch advocate of vaccination, White has seen a dramatic rise in childhood behavioral problems in her school district, as well as asthma, diabetes, and other chronic diseases, ever since the Hepatitis B vaccination was mandated for infants in 1991 [White]. Autism and other behavioral problems have also been linked to the DPT vaccine (for diphtheria, pertussis, tetanus), because of convulsions or cerebral inflammation that occurred hours or days after administration of the vaccine [Coulter90]. More recently, the MMR vaccine (for measles, mumps, rubella) has been implicated in an English study by Andrew Wakefield, MD [Wakefield]. This vaccine is suspected to cause abnormal intestinal problems in autistic children, and it is also suspected as a trigger for Crohn's disease. Although Wakefield's work has met with the criticism that one would expect for such an unpopular scientific result, his suspicions about the MMR vaccine have been buttressed by other studies. For example, American researcher V. K. Singh has found evidence that autism may be an autoimmune disorder of the brain that is triggered by the MMR vaccine [Singh]. Today, many parents within the American and British autism communities feel that this vaccine, in particular, is the culprit for their children's condition. I have come to believe that this was the case for Max as well.

It will be a shocking and sad day when we as a society admit to ourselves that, in our effort to avoid the childhood illnesses (many of which are usually benign) or to needlessly protect newborn infants from diseases primarily found among intravenous drug users (Hepatitis B), we may be inadvertently crippling many of our children, both mentally and physically, for life.

Luckily, homeopathy has a long-standing and successful track record in repairing vaccination damage. It also has been successful in curing (not just palliating) the allergies, asthma, and behavioral problems that may result from this damage. Max's story is a case in point. Homeopathic remedies are also available for treating and preventing the very same childhood diseases that vaccinations are trying to prevent. Thus, homeopathy provides not only a remedial tool but also an alternative way to achieve disease prevention.

THE PATH TO CURE

Max's cure was a miracle. There is still not a day that goes by without my thanking God for it. But Max's healing was not without its ups and downs. Invariably, overcoming a serious problem like autism is a process that takes time.

In retrospect, I realize that we were amazingly lucky to find a perfect remedy for Max right away. Because we were able to see at least some form of progress throughout Max's healing, it was easy to stick with the process. More often than not, however, it takes time for a homeopath to find a good remedy for a patient. This is especially true in complex, chronic cases. The net effect can be a sort of zigzag path to cure, a gradual and more circuitous return to health. After all, a homeopath can do nothing more than try to match a patient's current symptoms to the best fitting remedy they can find.

Of course, there are times when a quick miraculous cure does happen. I've seen it myself. I've already described some amazing cures that have occurred within my own family, especially in cases of acute disease. For example, I have seen a slowly rising fever, which had continued for several hours, stop dead in its tracks and resolve completely within a half hour after a remedy was taken. I have also seen an inflamed and painful welt from a wasp sting disappear in just a few minutes. A friend of mine was once prescribed a single low-potency dose of a remedy to help her back pain. It must have been the simillimum. Within the next couple of months, her rosacea (a skin problem that had troubled her for many years) completely resolved, she was able to go off her antidepressants, and her back pain resolved too!

But often, the path to cure is not so smooth. There may be periods of aggravation to deal with and modifications of dose and remedy to be tried. It takes patience, perseverance, and enough education about homeopathy to cooperate effectively with the treating homeopath and to cope with the bumps along the way.

Don't forget, a homeopath needs to know lots of symptoms — including some very personal ones — to make a good prescription. Without fully understanding a person's physical, mental, and emotional state, a homeopath can work only on the surface and can have only a superficial impact on a patient's health. Even when all of the relevant symptoms are known, it is often difficult to interpret a case correctly and find the simillimum. Because of this, the practice of homeopathy, like that of many other holistic healing therapies, is an art that requires years to master. In difficult cases, even the most experienced homeopath may need some time to understand a patient well enough to find a path to cure.

Another story from my own family might illustrate this point. My older son Izaak, a sensitive and intelligent child, suffered some ill-effects from our ordeal with Max. When he was seven (and Max was four), Izaak began to experience anxiety and tics. At times it was minor, but at times it was fairly severe. Of course, we also took him to John for treatment. But for a long time, nothing seemed to really work well or have a lasting effect.

At one point, Izaak's tics and twitches became so troublesome that I unilaterally gave him a dose of a remedy that is known as a "specific" for twitching. In other words, twitching is a prominent symptom associated with this remedy. The next morning, Izaak's tics were gone. Once again, it was a wonderful example of the rapid and dramatic effects that a remedy can have. But the prescription was superficial. It was based only upon Izaak's twitching, not on his overall state. Within a couple of weeks, the tics were back. And his anxieties were still there.

Over the next few years, we were eventually able to solve this puzzle and find some good remedies for Izaak. The first remedy that made a true impact on him was *Kali Bromatum* (potassium bromide). It is associated with an emotional feeling that one has caused or may cause some harm to a family member. One peculiar symptom of Kali Bromatum sums this up:

"Delusion, brother fell overboard in her sight."

In other words, the person feels as if he or she has witnessed an event like a sibling falling overboard from a boat. In truth, Izaak had deep feelings of responsibility for Max's problems. It is not uncommon for children to react this way to family troubles. Izaak's feelings were exacerbated by an actual event that literally mirrored the "falling overboard" symptom. In the summer of 1994, when we were visiting a large hotel, Max and Izaak ran down the hall to push the button for the elevator. Max got there first, pushed the button, and much to Izaak's horror, got onto the elevator alone. The doors closed before Izaak's eyes. We quickly got on the next elevator and took it down to the lobby, hoping Max had gone there as well. But he was nowhere to be found. I ran up and down the nine floors of the hotel and couldn't find him. Steve ran around outside the building. Izaak stood alone and helpless, waiting obediently in the lobby as we had asked him to do. Finally, after about 15 anxious minutes, hotel security found Max in the basement in the laundry room. Oddly, the basement was accessible only with a special elevator key. To this day, we still don't know how Max got there.

This event was extremely traumatic to Izaak, and he talked about it for many years. Whenever he thought Max might run off and get lost, Izaak would go into a panic. He also extended the same anxiety to our dog, needlessly worrying about her running away. Despite years of discussing this issue with him, Izaak continued to be anxious. But finally, after taking Kali Bromatum, he was able to leave these concerns behind. And his tics abated — in fact, they never became quite so severe again. Now, Kali Bromatum is *not* a common remedy for tics. But it is a remedy that touched the core of his anxiety.

Since then, Izaak has taken a few other remedies associated with similar emotional symptoms. Each has served to increasingly diminish his tendency toward anxiety. The next remedy we tried was *Cocculus Indicus*, the Indian cockle flower. It is well known for the treatment of people who are exhausted from nursing other family members and who tend to be overanxious about the health of others. I myself have also greatly benefited from this remedy. Another remedy that has helped Izaak is *Argentum Nitricum* (silver nitrate). Rajan Sankaran, one of the world's most eminent homeopaths and teachers from India, writes the following about this commonly used remedy:

> "It is a compound of silver (Ag) or Argentum, whose main theme is performance, and Nitrate, whose main theme is the feeling of sudden danger. The two come together in Argentum Nitricum, whose main theme is "Performance in sudden danger or crisis." There is a feeling as if the person will be accepted only if he can perform at the time of crisis." [Sankaran97, p. 16]

I have often felt that this must be exactly how Izaak felt as he anxiously stood and waited in the lobby of that hotel. Izaak's general level of anxiety about schoolwork and life in general has decreased considerably since taking this remedy. And, much to my own amazement, soon after taking his first dose, a few troublesome warts dried up and fell off.

THE MANY LESSONS LEARNED

Since I first published my original paper about Max's cure in 1998 [Lansky], I have been contacted by many parents of autistic children from around the world. Recently, one parent called to tell me that because of this paper, he had sought out homeopathic treatment for his autistic son — and that his boy was now recovering. That one phone call made all of my efforts to spread the word about Max's case worthwhile.

However, in most of my conversations with these beleaguered parents, I have discovered a great deal of resignation and fatalism about their child's condition. Despite my spending hours on the phone or E-mail with them, assuring them that autism had been cured in Max's case and had been treated successfully in other cases as well [HerscuAut], most of these parents have not given homeopathy a thorough trial. In one case, a mother sought out a homeopath and got a remedy for her child, but was too afraid to give it to her. In other cases, parents discontinued treatment after only a month, either because they didn't see enough effects from the remedy, or because they were scared by aggravations.

From these experiences I have learned the proverbial lesson — "You can lead a horse to water but you can't make him drink." It is my hope that, in the case of humans at least, further education can lead to an awareness of the need to take that first sip and keep drinking.

If someone comes to a homeopath because they are suffering from a chronic illness, they must give the homeopath time — at least six months — to find a good remedy and dosing regimen. Indeed, if an allopathic doctor has said that a condition is incurable, why are people surprised or discouraged when they are not cured quickly and easily by a homeopath? So often people turn to alternatives like homeopathy when all hope is lost, and they expect a miraculous cure to happen overnight. But cure usually takes time.

It also takes confidence. In the case of autism and other severe child-hood diseases, parents often become afraid and despondent, and under-standably so. It is hard enough for them to truly accept their child's illness. It is even harder for them to cultivate an attitude of confidence and trust that their child will be cured. In many cases, it is also difficult for them to face the potential disappointment of failed treatment. But what is worse? Disappointment, or a lifetime of caring for a child with a crippling disability?

I believe that it is an attitude of loving acceptance coupled with con-fidence in cure that is the key to recovery for anyone. I have read that it is not the fighters who recover from cancer. Rather, it is those individ-uals who are able to embrace their illness and its gifts, while still main-taining confidence that they will get to the other side of it. A difficult state of mind to achieve — no doubt about it! While acceptance of dis-ease may be achieved by some, if it is not coupled with confidence in cure, it can sometimes lead to psychological investment in disease. When this happens, the positive intentionality that fosters the curative process becomes derailed.

For example, I have met parents who have convinced themselves that their children are just fine being autistic. While this attitude may help a parent feel better about their situation, it does nothing to help a child recover. Certainly, their child would be better off if they weren't autis-tic. If we want our children (or ourselves) to recover, it is imperative that our love and acceptance be coupled with an inner vision of recovery. I believe this coupling of attitudes can be the single most powerful force in achieving a cure — the second most powerful, of course, being an accurately prescribed homeopathic remedy.

Being a homeopathic patient is invariably a journey of growth. It is a transformation, not a Band-Aid; a fulfillment of potential and a return to proper function, not a cut-and-paste operation. It may take effort, but cure (rather than unending palliation or suppression) is worth that effort. It takes awareness of one's symptoms and a willingness to divulge all aspects of oneself to a homeopath. It takes a "stick with it" attitude.

I hope that Max's story has also illustrated another point — the need to accommodate to improvement and growth as it occurs. Because a person undergoing homeopathic treatment may actually change in fundamental ways, it is important to make lifestyle modifications that accommodate that change. In a child's case, this may require changes in schooling or child-care arrangements. In an adult, the movement toward health may require changes in work or relationships. After all, in order to really heal, a person must often repair those circumstances that contribute to their illness.

Finally, homeopathy is ideally a family affair. For one thing, the healing of a child may actually depend on a parent's ability to change and become well too. Likewise, the healing of a child may free up family energy so that other family members can fulfill their own potential. In the end, homeopathy can improve the whole dynamic of a family, as a cycle of change and growth is set into motion. In our family, once Max was better, Steve and I were able to work on ourselves and our marriage. Eventually, Izaak was enabled to express his needs and have them addressed too. And the cycle still continues. I hope that my telling you about our experiences will help you, your family, and our society and world at large to find true healing. Because cure *is* possible.

CHAPTER 4

𝓎

WHAT IS DISEASE?
WHAT IS CURE?

"We see disease as the disattunement of the dynamis [vital force] — which will show up in the person not merely in one locale, but may manifest in diverse manners that may not seem to be related to each other from the perspective of reductionist pathology. As such, a person presenting with... athlete's foot, gastroesophageal reflux, and headache may have three 'diseases' according to allopathic nosology; but for us, there is likely one 'disease of the person' manifesting simultaneously in these three diverse superficial expressions. Homeopathy addresses the individual case of disease as it manifests diversely in the whole person, rather than pathologically-defined diseases as things in themselves."

— WILL TAYLOR, MD, 1999 [WT2]

THE BODY MACHINE

Fundamental to modern allopathic medicine is the view of the human body as an elaborate biochemical machine. Over time, our understanding of this machine has become more and more refined. With enough scrutiny, medical scientists hope to uncover every mechanism and detail of the human operating system. They have made great strides and the results have been truly impressive.

Because this model is so popular, most people believe that altering or tweaking components of the body machine will be enough to repair its faulty operation. The hope is that, just like an auto mechanic or a plumber, a doctor will be able to cure us by sealing off a leaky pipe here, removing a flawed part there, or by pouring in some chemical additives to increase operating efficiency.

As our understanding of the body has expanded, it has also become necessary for doctors to specialize in its subsystems. It has simply become impossible for any one person to achieve complete expertise on the whole machine. A side effect of this partitioning of expertise is the common belief that the body is partitioned in the same way. Thus, many people believe that their headaches have no relationship to their indigestion, or that their skin has no relationship to their respiratory system. Certainly applying cortisone cream to eczema couldn't lead to asthma?

But a plumber knows that sealing off a pipe will add pressure to the rest of a plumbing system. And a car mechanic knows that plugging up an exhaust valve or pouring some ill-advised additives into a gas tank will cause problems down the line. Caution is certainly even more warranted in the case of the human body. We are not machines. We are dynamic, integrated, and elaborate living entities.

Indeed, the results of a partitioned view of the body can be deadly. All too often we hear about someone who is taking 10 medications prescribed by 10 specialists for 10 different problems, and as a result is suffering from untold side effects and interactions. Below is a not atypical list of medications that was taken daily by a 55-year-old woman with chronic back pain:

Kapanol (morphine sulfate for back pain)
Prozac (antidepressant)
Premarin (hormone replacement)
Lipitor (for lowering cholesterol)
Diaformin (antidiabetic)
Prinvil (antihypertensive)
Quinate (for night cramps)
Losec (antiulcer/reflux)
Urocarb (urinary retention)
Uremide (diuretic)
Alodorm (for sleep)

Can anyone truly claim that such a drugging regimen is safe? For some people, just going off their numerous daily medications could bring total relief to a body spinning downward, out of control. Such people are the victims of *iatrogenic disease* — i.e., disease caused by pre-scribed medication and treatment. As mentioned in Chapter 2, this kind of disease is now estimated to be the third or fourth leading cause of death in America [Lazarou, Starfield] — far more than the number of deaths from car accidents. Going to yet another specialist to scrutinize yet another broken part of your body may be more dangerous to your health than getting onto the highway.

Jan Scholten, MD, a Dutch homeopath, has pointed out that allo-pathic and homeopathic diagnosis seem to stand at "right angles" to one another. The allopath sees and treats supposedly unrelated fragments of disease — eczema, pneumonia, an ulcer, depression. To a homeopath, these are only pieces of the overall pattern of a single underlying disease state. Scholten writes:

> "The difference between homoeopathic and allopathic diagnosis is sim-ilar to the sort of difference between pattern and grade, between form and size, between tone and volume. Allopathic medicine is concerned with measuring, whilst homoeopathy is concerned with shapes and patterns... Nearly every allopathic diagnosis is not a diagnosis at all in homoeopathic terms... The diagnosis of 'bronchitis' is only the begin-ning of a diagnosis in homoeopathic terms. We could compare this to the diagnosis of 'fever' in the middle ages. At that time fever was a real diagnosis which told you exactly what the patient was suffering from, whilst to us this sounds absurd. This is because we are so used to think-ing: 'Where does this fever come from?'... This example may illustrate that the concept 'diagnosis' implies the feeling 'I understand, so I don't have to look further.' This same situation exists in our present times with regard to a diagnosis of bronchitis, rheumatoid arthritis, myoma, colitis ulcerosa, etc. They are not real diagnoses, merely descriptions or syndromes. Homoeopathically speaking, this is only the start of the whole process of diagnosis, i.e., what is the remedy that belongs to this state? In fact we might say that in homoeopathic terms, the concepts 'disease,' 'diagnosis,' and 'remedy' are all one." [Scholten, pp. 830–831]

Rather than diagnose and treat the various parts of a disease, a homeopath will try to understand its overall pattern — composed of *all* of its symptoms, in every area of the body and mind. Once a homeopath has understood this pattern, he or she can try to match it to the pattern of a known remedy. And by giving this homeopathic or similarly pat- terned remedy, the homeopath treats the whole person — i.e., *treats all symptoms at once.*

It may seem incredible that a single substance could potentially cure all of our symptoms — our headaches, our depression, our indigestion and constipation, and our high blood pressure. But the holistic nature of homeopathic cures are illustrated daily in every homeopath's practice. Indeed, it is quite rare for a remedy to cure only one part of a person. If a remedy is truly curative, its effects usually extend to the whole person — because the remedy's symptoms match the whole person as well. In the following illustrative example, American professional homeopath Steve Waldstein, RSHom (NA), describes his own cure:

> "When I was given my first homeopathic remedy 25 years ago, my chief complaint was bronchitis lasting four months, leading to cracking ribs with coughing. The result of this remedy was: (1) The bronchitis went away immediately; (2) Asthma and allergies went away; (3) Emotionally, gigantic improvement; and (4) Moderate scoliosis that I had for 13 years — resulting in me spending a number of my teenage years in a back brace — disappeared over the next six months. It is amazing how deep the changes from the correct remedy can be." [SW1]

Steve also describes the case of one of his patients:

> "75-year-old with ulcerative colitis, osteoarthritis (one knee has been replaced and the other is looking bad), myocardial infarction and aneurism in past, hearing getting quite bad (wears hearing aid), emo- tionally no big problems (though the emotional state was the main thing leading to the prescription)... With aqueous doses of [remedy] over 18 months... The ulcerative colitis is almost totally gone — he still has a bit of urgency but only four bowel movements a day instead of 10–15, and always has time to make it to the bathroom. Colonoscopy shows no problem at all anymore. Hearing — dramatically better.

Osteoarthritis — no longer any problem with other knee. Blood pressure — down. Blood chemistry much better (despite no change in diet). Much happier." [SW2]

In other words, a true homeopathic cure is *systemic*. Rather than patching or repairing a part of the body, a curative remedy can bring about a widespread restoration of health to the entire organism — a fundamental change of state that addresses the true root of a patient's disease.

WE ARE MORE THAN MACHINES

"In the healthy human state, the spirit-like life force... that enlivens the material organism as dynamis, governs without restriction and keeps all parts of the organism in admirable, harmonious, vital operation, as regards both feelings and functions, so that our indwelling, rational spirit can freely avail itself of this living, healthy instrument for the higher purposes of our existence." [Hahnemann, Aphorism 9]

The limitations of the body-machine model and the folly of piecemeal treatment of individual symptoms becomes even more apparent if we accept the idea that there is more to us than just our physical body. Allopathic medicine is nearly alone among the world's medicines in its insistence that bodily disease is completely physical. What if modern allopathy is wrong and Indian, Chinese, and other medicines (including homeopathy) are right? If so, our physical body is merely a veneer or surface view of an elaborate and dynamic energetic entity — an entity that Hahnemann called the *dynamis* or *vital force*. This force incorporates our bodies, emotions, mind, and spirit, and interacts in inexplicable ways with other people, animals, plants, minerals, and even man-made creations. Perhaps one day we may develop sophisticated instruments for detecting and measuring the vital force. But for now, all we can do is observe how it manifests itself in terms of physical and behavioral symptoms, and try to find reliable methods for working with it. Certainly, accepting the reality of such a force changes the whole medical equation.

Of course, many allopathic doctors have begun to acknowledge that disease may extend beyond the physical — that a person's emotions and thoughts can interact with their physical body. For example, most people today acknowledge that life's stresses can affect blood pressure, bring out eczema, or trigger asthmatic attacks. But the growing allopathic understanding of holism is still quite partial and superficial. Although allopaths acknowledge that there may be mind-body connections, most believe that these connections are strictly biochemical. It must be neurohormones at work. It must be a brain chemical imbalance that's causing our depression. The response: prescribe antidepressants or megadoses of vitamins — pour in some more additives.

But the body keeps breaking down — and we keep patching, adding, and cutting. We invent new drugs, but bacteria and viruses mutate and keep up. We dump in new vaccinations, but new and stronger diseases arise. We take antidepressants, but are we really happy, deep down inside? In the meantime, our bodies and minds are becoming weakened by all of these things. Our inherent susceptibility to disease has become greater. The signs are everywhere. Just look around you. Even children have become the victims of severe chronic diseases at rates much higher than was true in the past.

These trends should be causing alarm bells to go off in our society. And, indeed, some allopaths have begun to be concerned. For, despite our increasingly technological medical capabilities, the tools available for treating chronic disease are actually fairly limited in scope. The result is a kind of desperation in conventional medicine today. But rather than genuinely looking "outside the box" for true alternatives, the natural tendency for most allopaths is to believe that developing more drugs, vaccines, and surgical procedures will eventually overcome something they do not understand very well at all.

For instance, consider the modern practice of prophylactic hysterectomies. These are sometimes recommended for symptom-free young women if their family medical history indicates a strong tendency towards uterine or ovarian cancer. But does removing a woman's organs also remove her inherent tendency to develop cancer? If a body copes with life stresses by developing cancer, won't it simply develop cancer in some other organ? And does this woman even have the tendency to develop cancer? What will be the untoward effects of removing key hormone-producing organs from her body? What happens to her if she is given hormone replacement therapy, a treatment already known to increase the chances of developing cancer?

In my view, a wiser approach would be to try to remove or reduce this woman's *susceptibility* to cancer. The way to achieve this can be found by adopting an alternative medical view — that susceptibility resides in the energy body, not in the physical body-machine.

A fundamental discovery of 20th century physics was that the building blocks of our reality are much more subtle than they appear to be. True reality is at the quantum level, where thoughts can have effects, and events and actions do not have to be physically close to one another in order to interact. Clearly, modern medicine has not kept up with these discoveries. It is still operating from a Newtonian premise: that the human body — surely one of the most subtle and complex systems that exists — is a big plumbing system. Modern medicine has yet to incorporate the scientific outlook of the 20th century.

Amazingly, Hahnemann, even at the turn of the 19th century, was able to come up with a radically different and intrinsically energetic viewpoint: that the physical body is coupled to an invisible vitalistic force that is the true organizing principle of life. Certainly, his successful use of ultradilute remedies reinforced this view. But what really enabled Hahnemann to make such a cognitive leap was a philosophical shift. Rather than trying to develop a new, more complex model of the body machine, Hahnemann's response to the medical predicament of his time was to rethink everything. In particular, he accepted as a premise that a complete understanding of how the body functions was impossible, and that, in fact, *this understanding was not necessary for the successful practice of medicine*. As a result, he was freed up to find a system of medicine that did not depend on this understanding.

Of course, this seems odd to those of us with a mechanistic view of the body. Surely, you can't fix something unless you know exactly how it works. But what if you *can't* completely know how something works? In this situation, you will focus on empirical observation and experience — in the case of medicine, on what seems to consistently heal or improve the body's functioning. Moreover, your fundamental research goal will be different. *You will try to determine what actually cures, rather than figure out how the body works.* And through your experiments, you may eventually derive principles or laws about the relationship between curative agents and the diseases they cure.

This is precisely what Hahnemann did. He focused on what actually cured — not on what seemed logical from the perspective of a particular model of the body — and ultimately he discovered a general-purpose law of cure, the Law of Similars. When he applied this principle, he met with great success.

WE ARE INTRINSICALLY SELF-HEALING

In Chapter 2, we discussed how Hahnemann was a naturalist when it came to health, even before he discovered the Law of Similars. To him it was plain common sense that the body is dynamic and integrated, and that when left to its own devices, it will usually be able to repair itself. We are animals after all, just like other animals on this planet, and we are probably even better equipped to adapt and survive. Surely we must have evolved to be self-repairing, self-healing. Our bodies have built-in mechanisms to maintain balance, even in the face of physical and emotional challenges.

Unfortunately, a trust in the body's inherent wisdom and strength seems to have been lost in the modern world. So many of us think of ourselves as flawed, fragile, disconnected machines. We think we need all kinds of props to hold us up. "I have a brain chemical deficiency." "I need more hormones." "I need antidepressants." This view is a modern creation, an illusion we have all bought into, largely due to the influence of the powerful medical and advertising industries. For thousands of years, our ancestors had no access to antibiotics, antidepressants, or antihistamines. Surely the human body is not as frail as we think.

Of course, sometimes the external forces of life do become too much for us. In response, we develop a state of being that is not perfectly balanced; we become skewed. Perhaps our lungs become a weak spot. Perhaps a difficult childhood leaves us prone to anxiety or paranoia. Once we become skewed enough, we tend to become more severely ill as difficult situations arise. Minor illnesses take longer to recover from. We become more allergic and sensitive to our environment. What began as minor spells of the blues becomes a chronic state of depression.

But even if someone is in a chronic state of disease, it is important to remember that they are not without defenses. Within all of our bodies are mechanisms whose entire purpose is to maintain life, heal our wounds, and reachieve balance. All parts of the body are interrelated and working together to create the best possible adaptation to every circumstance. How can we enhance these mechanisms rather than supplant them with chemicals? One way to regain and enhance this ability for self-repair is via homeopathic treatment. Somehow, a properly selected remedy functions as an energetic stimulus or information transmitter that enables the body to do what it has forgotten or become less able to do: heal itself.

SYMPTOMS ARE OUR FRIENDS

"Disease is a unit. It is one disease for one person at one time. It begins in a single place (usually the individual's weakest spot) but it also shows itself throughout the whole being in many ways, manifesting though many signposts which we call signs and symptoms. Our job is to ferret out that ONE disease for that one person. The vital force's job is to help us find it, by producing signs, or symptoms, that show us the pattern of the disease." [Herscu, p. 6]

So what about disease? What about those nasty symptoms? Once you believe that the body and mind are always doing their best to accommodate to every situation, symptoms take on a whole new meaning and significance:

Symptoms are usually manifestations of the body's best attempt to heal itself. This view of symptoms may seem odd at first. After all, machines can't repair themselves. When our car breaks down, its "symptoms" aren't signs of self-repair — they are signs of disrepair. But the body is not a machine. It does repair itself. We would all die quite rapidly if this were not the case. Thus, when we develop a fever or vomit, it is usually because the body is trying to kill off invading bacteria or purge itself of toxic matter. When we become hysterical or depressed after an emotional incident, it is the psyche's way of coping and healing from that incident. Symptoms, especially in acute disease, are signs that our defensive system is working.

Consider this. If we did not develop symptoms — if we did not develop a fever when it was warranted or become upset after a traumatic event — we would be quite sick indeed. When a person cannot develop symptoms, it is a sign that their inherent vitality is quite weak. We all know that elderly people do not usually develop high fevers as children do. This is because a young child has a good vital reactive system; a child can develop a high fever that enables them to quickly heal. An older person can only put up a weaker defense, and as a result, it is much harder for them to get well.

Now, if a symptom is a sign of the body's attempt to heal, what are the consequences of suppressing it? What if we suppress every fever with aspirin and every rash with cortisone? Palliate every allergic reaction with antihistamines? Quell every depression with antidepressants? This has become the primary operative mode of modern allopathic medicine — temporarily palliation or complete suppression of symptoms. But what is the effect of this practice in the long run — or even in the short-term?

Consider the use of nasal decongestant spray. Such sprays only temporarily alleviate congestion, they do not cure it. The congestion always returns after the spray wears off. Indeed, we are warned not to use such sprays for too long; if we do, our congestion will become even worse. This phenomenon illustrates a more general point. If we palliate or keep pushing our symptoms down, the body will rebel. It wants those symptoms. If you push them down, they will come back with a vengeance, or perhaps pop up somewhere else, in some other form.

Now what if you go beyond palliation and succeed in completely suppressing a symptom? A recent television ad for herpes medication enthusiastically exclaims, "It's all about suppression!" If you artificially suppress a symptom so that it never reappears, you may have the illusion of cure. But in reality, the underlying disease state that is causing that symptom will have to find a different way to express itself. Don't forget, if the body's symptoms reflect its battle against disease — a battle that is being waged in the most benign way possible — then its symptoms will usually be ones that are least damaging to health, given the circumstances. After all, the body's underlying "goal" is to survive. But if we completely deny and suppress these symptoms, the body will eventually need to compensate — by expressing itself with more serious symptoms elsewhere.

Hahnemann began to witness this phenomenon early on in his career. One of his first observations about disease was that it tended to deepen after suppressive treatments. This was particularly obvious when skin symptoms were suppressed. For instance, Hahnemann noticed that suppressed eczema could lead to asthma and other respiratory problems. The same observation can be made today. Modern pediatricians have all witnessed the rise of allergies and asthma in children, and they usually assume that pollution is the culprit. But what if the true culprit is the overuse of cortisone and allergy medicines? The following message, posted to a homeopathy Internet list by a concerned parent, provides a typical example of this syndrome:

> "My 17-month-old daughter is suffering from "childhood eczema" (as diagnosed by her pediatrician). We have used "1% Hydrocortisone"... ointment when needed, up to twice a day. The medication usually helps, but is not a cure for the eczema which began during the first month or so after birth. This was also when she received the first of many vaccinations required or recommended in Illinois where we live...
>
> My older daughter who is now nine used to have the same problem. Her eczema went away around age four, but was replaced by occasional asthma attacks. The asthma attacks now occur only once or twice a year. I have severe pollen allergies. My wife has mild pollen allergies. I hope this information helps." [MC]

From the homeopathic point of view, a weak spot in this family's health pattern is the tendency to develop eczema, allergies, and asthma. The children both developed eczema early on, perhaps as a reaction to vaccination. When their eczema was suppressed, their underlying disease tendency was forced to express itself as asthma.

CURE VERSUS SUPPRESSION

After Hahnemann recognized the effects of symptom suppression, he began to examine more deeply the links between disease episodes, and especially, the effects of homeopathic remedies on symptom progression. He found that if symptoms were treated and removed homeopathically, *they would be cured without further progression of disease.* Moreover, *earlier symptoms that had once been suppressed would return.* Thus, if a case of asthma was cured homeopathically, the eczema that preceded the asthmatic state would most likely return. And if the eczema was then cured homeopathically (rather than suppressed), there would no longer be a progression into asthma.

Hahnemann also noticed proof of this in nature. He discovered that when disease episodes were left completely untreated and proceeded naturally, their interrelationships and patterns of progression and recession would reflect the same phenomena. For example, Hahnemann observed that if a patient was suffering from a disease and then contracted another *dissimilar* disease on top of it, the first disease would often disappear; it would become temporarily suppressed. However, once the second disease resolved, the first disease would return. This pattern mirrors the use of palliative drug treatment. Hahnemann wrote:

> "When measles and smallpox were reigning at the same time, and both infected the same child, the measles that had already broken out was usually halted in its course by the smallpox that broke out somewhat later. The measles did not resume its course until after the smallpox healed." [Hahnemann, Aphorism 38]

I've even seen this phenomenon myself. Izaak had a mild nose cold and cough that disappeared completely when he contracted a 24-hour stomach flu. When the flu resolved, the cold returned.

A second kind of disease combination that Hahnemann observed is analogous to the use of homeopathic remedies. In this case, the second disease is *similar* to the first. The result is that when the second disease resolves, the first disease resolves as well and never returns. For example, Hahnemann made this observation about the two similar diseases cowpox and smallpox — indeed, at about the same time as Edward Jenner did. Jenner's observation led him to the use of cowpox as a vaccination for smallpox. Hahnemann's observations and conclusions ran deeper. He noticed that incurring and recovering from smallpox could also cure deafness, testicular swelling, and dysentery that also just happened to precede it. He realized that this happened because all of these symptoms were also characteristic of smallpox; i.e., the process of getting and recovering from smallpox enabled the cure of previously existing conditions whose symptoms were similar to those of smallpox. Hahnemann also understood that Jenner's successful use of cowpox as a vaccination for smallpox was merely an illustration of a much larger therapeutic principle — the Law of Similars. (Nevertheless, as will be discussed later on, the way vaccination is practiced by allopaths is very much at odds with homeopathic philosophy and practice; the homeopathic approach to prophylaxis against disease is quite different.)

Finally, Hahnemann also observed cases in which two dissimilar diseases combined and coexisted. This was particularly common when a natural disease combined with an *iatrogenic* disease — a disease caused by toxic doses of medicine. Hahnemann noticed that iatrogenic diseases tend to persist and ultimately coexist with a patient's original disease. In modern times, this can be seen in people whose symptoms are suppressed with ongoing use of steroids; ultimately, the patient develops a "steroid disease" that coexists with their original illness.

Because of these observations, Hahnemann came to view the effects of all medicines as diseases in themselves. A "medicinal disease" could be viewed as either similar or dissimilar to a patient's disease. Eventually, Hahnemann concluded that the only way to cure a disease — not palliate or suppress it — was to meet it with a similar medicinal disease. In other words, the only way to cure was homeopathically.

ANTIPATHY, HOMEOPATHY, AND ALLOPATHY

Hahnemann's observations about the various possible relationships between disease states and medicinal states are fundamental to understanding the difference between homeopathy and other forms of medicine. Indeed, it was Hahnemann who coined the terms *allopathy*, *antipathy*, and *homeopathy*, in order to distinguish among different ways of applying medicines to diseases.

- *Anti-pathy* is the application of medicines according to what Hippocrates called the *Law of Opposites*. In other words, to counter a symptom, a medicine is given that, if it were given to a healthy person, would create the opposite effect of the symptom. For example, a drying agent might be used in cases of excess mucus, or a constipating agent might be used for diarrhea.

- *Homeo-pathy* is the application of medicines to disease states according to the *Law of Similars*. In other words, to cure a symptom, a medicine is given that, in a healthy person, would bring about a similar symptom.

- *Allo-pathy* is the application of medicines to disease states according to no particular rule or law. In other words, the effects of medicines on healthy people bears no fixed relationship to their use in sick people. An allopathic physician may make use of antipathic medicines, homeopathic medicines, or any other kind of medicinal substance or method; there is no guiding principle of therapeutics.

Given the above definitions, it is clear that antipathic medicines are primary tools of today's allopaths. This is reflected in their use of antidepressants, antihistamines, antiinflammatories, etc. From the standpoint of homeopathic philosophy, all uses of antipathy are either palliative (i.e., they merely suppress a symptom for a short time, after which it returns) or are completely suppressive (they permanently suppress a symptom at the risk of developing deeper disease later on).

Interestingly, some of today's allopathic treatments are homeopathic. For example, the heart medications nitroglycerin and digitalis are both tried-and-true homeopathic remedies that were used by homeopaths in the 1800s for cardiovascular disease. Because of the success of these remedies, they were adopted by the allopaths and continue to be used for heart patients until this day.

Of course, when modern allopaths discover new drugs that happen to have homeopathic action, they are puzzled. For instance, doctors are puzzled why Ritalin, a stimulant, should have a calming effect on hyperactive children. Of course, I'm not suggesting Ritalin as an effective homeopathic cure for hyperactivity. From a homeopathic perspective, Ritalin is applied in a blanket, nonindividualized fashion, and is given in toxic doses. But the reason why it works at all is due to the homeopathic principle — likes cure likes. Another somewhat amusing example of this phenomenon appeared in a recent article in the *Houston Chronicle*:

> " An intriguing new study suggests coffee may prevent Parkinson's disease. How a product that makes people jittery could keep them from getting a disease that gives them tremors is not examined... but ... the study found that men who didn't drink coffee were five times more likely to develop Parkinson's than those who drank the most." [HoustonChronicle]

Once again, heavy coffee drinking is not a recommended habit for anyone, but its ability to prevent or reduce the incidence of Parkinson's disease may also be explained by the Law of Similars.

Allopathic medicines that are neither antipathic nor homeopathic are actually considered the most dangerous by homeopaths. They are so strong that they completely suppress symptoms by engrafting a new, stronger medicinal disease onto a patient. The result is that patients now have two diseases — a disguised but deepened version of their original disease (which will most likely take on a new form) and an iatrogenic disease caused by the medicine. Typical examples of this kind of therapy are the use of chemotherapy for cancer and psychotropic medications for the severely mentally ill.

Over the past two hundred years, the Law of Similars has proven to be a therapeutic strategy that consistently cures without suppression. It may seem unbelievable, but it is true; homeopathic medicines can cure supposedly incurable conditions like asthma — conditions that allopaths can only palliate or suppress. And, when properly applied, homeopathic remedies do not engraft new disease states. Indeed, they have the power to reveal previous layers of disease that were suppressed before, thereby allowing for their homeopathic treatment as well.

Of course, in serious cases, especially when many allopathic drugs have been taken over a long period of time, complete homeopathic cure can be long and complex — sometimes impossible. The curative process may require expert monitoring and care from both an experienced homeopath and an allopathic physician, to enable gradual and safe weaning off allopathic drugs. But if the body is able, such cures do happen. And even if complete cure is not possible, most people can attain a significant improvement in their health and a decrease in their need for allopathic medication.

One final word of caution. Just because a medicine is ultradilute and potentized does not make its use homeopathic. Potentized medicines can be applied antipathically and allopathically in the hands of a person who does not fully understand their use and cannot distinguish between suppression and cure. For this reason, remedies should always be used with caution, preferably under the supervision of a certified homeopath.

THE LAW OF CURE

As I have already described, Hahnemann's observational skills enabled him to recognize causal interrelationships between disease episodes. He also noticed that, depending on a person's particular susceptibilities and areas of weakness, his or her disease progression would usually take a fairly predictable path. Of course, allopaths have also noticed that people tend to manifest typical pathways of disease progression. But what about the reverse direction? What does a cure look like? And how can it be distinguished from suppression?

As I mentioned earlier, the successful homeopathic treatment of disease is often heralded by the reappearance of old symptoms. In essence, the progression toward deeper disease is put into reverse; the outermost disease state is met by a remedy and is lifted, revealing layers that had been suppressed before. These old symptoms can then be treated homeopathically, or, in many cases, do not need treatment at all — they simply "pass through" in lessened form and disappear by themselves. I have seen this in my own case. After taking a remedy, I experienced the return of precancerous cells on my nose that had been burned off years earlier. However, unlike before, these cells now scabbed over and healed completely on their own.

As it turns out, the old symptoms that return during a curative process tend to occur in a particular kind of pattern or sequence. Homeopaths call this pattern the *Law of Cure*. Although not a "law" like the Law of Similars, it can be viewed as an observational guideline for recognizing a pattern of cure, in contrast to a pattern of disease progression. The Law of Cure states that cure tends to proceed:

- *From the center toward the circumference.*
- *From above, downward.*
- *From more vital to less vital organs.*
- *In reverse order of appearance.*

Thus, internal (and more important) organs tend to be healed first, with the skin usually coming last. Symptoms also tend to return and be healed starting from the head and torso and progressing outward toward the limbs. Finally, symptoms tend to heal in reverse order of their appearance. Of course, this "top-down, in-out, last-first" pattern of cure isn't always strictly followed. The underlying idea, however, is that symptoms tend to be healed so that the most threatening symptoms are cured first. Since disease tends to progress by following the least harmful path of symptom expression, it also makes sense that the body will tend to heal its most important parts first.

The following case treated by Malaysian homeopath and physician Dr. Suriya Osman, illustrates the Law of Cure beautifully. It also demonstrates the dangers of suppression.

"This patient... was first seen in 1988 with what seemed to be a simple case of dandruff. He later developed tinea versicolor [a benign loss of pigmentation of the skin] both of which were treated in a suppressive manner. In 1991 this patient developed a full blown case of psoriasis with abdominal pain and also joint pain. He was referred to a skin specialist who put him on steroids and the usual skin creams... This patient had been on steroids, NSAID's [non-steroidal anti-inflammatory drugs] (Ponstan), and a paraphernalia of creams ever since, with a symptom picture getting worse and worse... In March of 1998, he complained of bodyache in addition to his usual joint pain and skin lesions. I looked over his records and was alarmed at the amount of steroids he had consumed. I asked if he would mind a slight aggravation and told him I was afraid that the steroids might have weakened his bones. I gave him [remedy] for a week hoping to antidote some of the bad effects of the steroids. I did not see this patient until today. He told me he had not taken any Ponstan ever since my treatment, had not needed any antihistamines and the only skin lesions he had were tinea versicolor! The remedy had brought back the old problem and miraculously taken away his joint pain, abdominal pain and psoriasis... The amazing thing is that the patient did not appear to realize that a near miracle had taken place! He did experience a very slight aggravation for about two days when he started the remedy, but has otherwise been well." [SO]

And a follow-up:

"The patient came back today because he had a slight cold and cough. I asked him about his psoriasis, to date, no symptoms at all. His skin still shows the tinea versicolor. His joint pains only come during wet weather and then only very slightly and only in the morning. I asked him about mental symptoms. While he used to be very easily irritated and angry, was anxious at night due to the pain from the joints, he is now an even tempered fellow who sleeps soundly all night. It still amazes me that all he needed was [remedy] for a week for a condition that spanned 10 years and was labeled incurable by our orthodox specialists!" [SO]

Notice how the treatment of this man's severe body pains (initially caused by suppression of skin disease, coupled with iatrogenic disease due to prolonged steroid use) led to a return of the original benign skin complaint of tinea versicolor. This case also illustrates how important it is not to suppress skin symptoms, including those that may reappear during the process of homeopathic cure. Such symptoms are typically not life-threatening and may indicate that deeper disease is simply on its way out. A homeopath should always be consulted if there is any question or doubt about returning symptoms. Remember that skin symptoms are often the body's best safety valve for venting disease. Unfortunately, in our vain and image-conscious society, they are also the first symptoms we suppress.

Here is another illustrative case that describes the retreat of Lyme disease. Notice how the disease regressed in the exact reverse order of its progression. The patient was treated by Christian Kurz, PhD, an Austrian nuclear physicist who is also a homeopath.

"A man came to me... with the diagnosis of Lyme disease. It was a textbook case, with the wandering exanthema [skin eruption] and accompanying pains. The skin symptoms had already subsided, and the muscle pains set in. They were so severe that the pain caused him to perspire so profusely that he would leave a little puddle wherever he was standing for a few minutes. He couldn't walk anymore and was sitting in a wheelchair. The pain had started in the area of the right forearm and had wandered up the arm, around the neck and had settled above the sternum on the chest... After the remedy, the pain retraced the original path. There was a hint of an exanthema on the original spot and all was over in a week. After one week he was completely restored and went on a trip to Bangkok. I have seen him several times since then (2.5 months ago) with no sign of recurrence." [CK]

Since homeopathy deals with the whole person, not just the physical body, the Law of Cure actually applies on a much deeper and more complete level than implied by these two cases. Even before remedies help to heal the physical body, they often address the innermost part of our being — our psyche, our mind, and our emotions. Thus, a common pattern of homeopathic cure begins with an increased sense of inner well-being. This may then be followed by healing on the physical level.

A classic example might be a lessening of anxiety, followed by a cure of asthma, followed by the return of eczema on the face. After this heals, the eczema might migrate out to the limbs, and then finally leave totally. In contrast, it would be a sign of suppression if asthma disappeared only to be replaced by new and more serious symptoms, such as severe depression or heart disease.

Homeopaths usually attribute the Law of Cure to Constantine Hering, MD, the first leader of the homeopathic community in America. A colorful and brilliant man, Hering was born in 1800 in Saxony, Germany. The pupil of the prominent surgeon Robbi at the University of Leipzig, he first came to homeopathy as a debunker; he was asked by his professors to write a paper condemning Hahnemann's new system. In his attempt to honestly do so, he repeated Hahnemann's original experiment with cinchona and found it to be successful. Shortly thereafter, he was cured of a potentially fatal dissecting wound with a single homeopathic dose of *Arsenicum Album* (arsenic trioxide). Soon he began to study and utilize the homeopathic system, and he quickly became an ardent supporter. As he himself wrote:

> "My enthusiasm grew. I became a fanatic. I went about the country, visited inns, where I got up on tables and benches to harangue whoever might be present to listen to my enthusiastic speeches on homeopathy. I told the people that they were in the hands of cut-throats and murderers. Success came everywhere. I almost thought I could raise the dead." [Knerr]

Hering arrived in America in 1833 and became the leader among the few homeopaths there at the time. He settled in Allentown, Pennsylvania, and started a homeopathic college in that city in 1837. Later, in 1844, he founded America's first medical society, the American Institute of Homeopathy.

Hering was an avid enthusiast of collecting symptoms that had not only appeared in provings, but had also been verifiably cured by remedies. Indeed, he published his own 10-volume materia medica, whose remedy symptoms are still considered some of the most reliable to this day. Hering was also an inveterate prover of new medicines. He proved more than 100 remedies on himself, including the snake remedy *Lachesis* (made from the poisonous venom of the bushmaster snake) and *Glonoine* — the medicine today known as nitroglycerin. As mentioned before, nitroglycerin is one of several homeopathic medicines that are still used by today's allopaths. Every heart patient with a little bottle of "nitro" under his or her pillow (my mother being one of them) owes a debt of thanks to Constantine Hering.

Unfortunately, knowledge of Hering's Law of Cure — simple yet critical observations about the signs of true cure — has yet to reach today's allopaths. Consider the following story from my own family. My older son Izaak had minor eczema as a baby, which we suppressed with cortisone cream. He then went on to develop allergies. As our pediatrician wrote out a prescription for allergy medicine, she commented, "He will probably develop asthma." Did she ever stop to think that the previous cortisone treatment had led to Izaak's allergies and that the suppressive allergy medicine she was prescribing might be the ultimate cause of asthma?

Doctors may notice that progressions tend to occur and that symptoms tend to become deeper and more significant, but they never ask why. It just happens. It's a "tendency." Yes, it's true that people have tendencies toward specific kinds of disease progressions. But because symptoms are routinely suppressed rather than treated homeopathically, doctors never get to see what a real cure looks like, with the return of older and lesser symptoms. They do not even know that such cures are possible.

Thankfully, we discontinued allergy medicines for Izaak, and he never developed asthma. He still suffers from some minor allergies, but he manages without antihistamines or any other kind of allergy medicine. He even has a bit of eczema return now and then. I am happy to see it! We just let it be, and eventually it resolves on its own or as a result of ongoing homeopathic treatment.

Another anecdote concerns a friend of mine. She has suffered for many years from respiratory problems, including asthma and bronchitis, which she routinely suppresses, mostly with over-the-counter medications. Because she cannot afford health insurance, she is forced to go to the emergency room in crises, where she is given antibiotics, steroids, and a growing stack of medical bills that she cannot afford to pay. Eventually, her condition worsened. Although she no longer had as many respiratory symptoms, she developed severe emotional agitation and chest pain and subsequently suffered several minor strokes. The medical bills racked up further. I could see she was in grave danger — at the age of 45. I helped her pay some of her medical bills and convinced my family homeopath to take her on without a fee. He was able to find a good remedy for her quickly. Her chest pains, headaches, and sleeplessness subsided considerably for the few months she stayed on the recommended remedy. However, her bronchial and asthma symptoms returned, which she soon suppressed. Months later, her heart problems returned as well. Unfortunately, I have not been able to convince her to return to the homeopath.

My friend's story is the story of many Americans. They cannot afford to take even a few days off from work in order to heal, nor can they afford health insurance or the services of a doctor that is able to follow their case carefully. In the end, they take too many ill-advised medications and develop even more serious chronic problems than most people do.

Homeopathy could be a cost-effective way to help the poor. Although the consultation rates are not inexpensive, the remedy costs are negligible and the results, in the long run, are more satisfactory and cost-effective. But the current legal status of homeopathic practice in this country, as well as the fact that it is not usually covered by insurance, makes treatment of the poor a risky and unviable option for most homeopaths. In addition, the "quick fix" mentality of most Americans makes homeopathic treatment problematic. Most people expect immediate results — usually immediate palliation or suppression — which homeopathy cannot always provide.

SUSCEPTIBILITY

So why *do* we get sick? From an allopathic standpoint — the one most of us were indoctrinated with — we are the victims of "germs." Those pesky bacteria and viruses are everywhere, lurking on every doorknob and stranger's hand. If we are unlucky and get attacked, we are their hapless victims.

But wait! That can't be the whole story. Not everyone exposed to a virus or bacteria gets sick. The kids may all get the cold going around, but the parents might not. And doctors don't get every disease they are exposed to; they know how to put up some kind of "energetic" barrier to disease, and it usually works. Besides, we know that germs are everywhere. There is no escaping them. If becoming sick were simply a matter of exposure, we would all be sick all of the time.

The fact is, a person isn't necessarily the victim of every bacterium that jumps into his or her nose. Even in the most virulent epidemic, not everyone gets sick or dies. Some people can swim in frigid lakes without getting sick; others fall ill when exposed to a cool breeze. Some people can endure gruesome abusive childhoods and come away stronger; others are left permanently scarred by comparatively mild upsets. It's all a matter of our individual *susceptibility* — our ability to defend ourselves, to regain and retain equilibrium in the face of the onslaughts of daily life. That's why a physically and mentally healthy person is able to deal with most bacteria, viruses, and the natural ups and downs of life without much help. After all, the human world is and always has been full of germs, pollution, poor foods, grief, fear, and poverty. There's no escaping it all, and no spray will sterilize sufficiently.

So if disease isn't simply and irrevocably caused by an enemy outside ourselves, what is the cause? The answer is that there are at least two forces at work: the external world of the environment and the internal world of the patient. If a patient falls sick, it is because the world has dealt them a blow *and* they were susceptible to it; their mind/body was simply not able to adapt and regain equilibrium. That is why homeopaths think the best defense is prevention: observing sound hygienic and dietary practices, and enhancing the body's physical and emotional ability to cope more effectively with whatever life does bring — i.e., decreasing susceptibility.

This is precisely what homeopathic treatment can do. Somehow, a remedy that is truly homeopathic to the state of a patient can not only cure them, but can also reduce their susceptibility and improve their ability to adapt and recover in general. For example, before undergoing homeopathic treatment several years ago, I was increasingly prey to every cold or flu going around. Each year, I found myself getting sick more and more often, and taking longer and longer to recover — often weeks. Today, I rarely get a cold — at most two or three times a year. When I do, it usually takes me only two or three days to recover — without the aid of any conventional medicine.

Of course, the allopathic model of disease treatment is quite different. Bacteria and viruses are cast as enemy agents and treatment as warfare. The result is a never-ending and often escalating series of battles. First there is the skirmish, where symptoms are patched over and suppressed. Then there is warfare — with ever-stronger drugs. We creep about stealthily, avoiding "the enemy" as much as possible. We spray each crevice with protective antibacterial soaps, or dose ourselves prophylactically with antibiotics. But unfortunately, these practices just serve to strengthen the bacteria that surround us, whether we like it or not; the enemy knows how to adapt.

The truth is, by avoiding all aggravating influences, we may actually be depriving ourselves of the opportunity to learn how to deal with them. For instance, if children are sheltered so completely that they never experience sadness, jealousy, or anger, they won't know how to operate very effectively when they leave the family nest. Likewise, if we suppress every disease and kill every germ artificially, our bodies won't learn how to deal with these disease factors on their own. Remember: people were once able to recover from many infections without antibiotics. We should be reserving our big guns for the real battles.

The same argument can be made about vaccination. Medical scientists are developing more and more types of vaccines against viruses each year. But invariably, new and more vicious diseases are discovered as well. While the goal of vaccination may be to stimulate the immune system, research has also shown that the immune mechanisms they create aren't exactly the same nor as beneficial as the mechanisms developed by actually contracting and recovering from a disease [Parish]. As discussed in the preceding chapter, vaccines boost the humoral or Th2 function of the immune system; actually getting (and recovering) from a disease boosts cell-mediated or Th1 immunity. To overstimulate one type of immunity at the expense of another may be ill-advised. Indeed, there is a very real possibility that overvaccination of today's children may be inadvertently triggering a variety of allergic and autoimmune disorders (because of overstimulation of the Th2 immune function). It may also be diminishing the ability of the Th1 immune functions to fight disease in general. As immunity researcher Philip F. Incao, MD, points out, "There is no system of the human being, from the mind to muscles to immune system, which gets stronger through avoiding challenges, but only through overcoming challenges. The wise use of vaccinations would be use them selectively, and not on a mass scale." [Incao]

As it turns out, the childhood diseases such as measles, mumps, and chicken pox used to be regarded as *beneficial* by pediatricians. Doctors of the past noticed that, after experiencing and recovering from these diseases, children tended to make developmental leaps in cognition and physical robustness. The natural experience of these childhood diseases may even be necessary for our children's normal development. They certainly do exercise the immune system and develop a natural and permanent form of immunity — something that cannot always be said of vaccinations. So what is the effect of removing these experiences from our children's lives?

Unfortunately, the rate of vaccine use is only accelerating. As recently as 1985, the recommended vaccination schedule in America delivered 25 antigens [disease agents] to children by the time they were five years old.

By 2002, that number had increased to 77 antigens [Mercola], and the numbers are increasing each year. Our societal reliance on vaccinations for every kind of virus may ultimately come at the cost of terrible side effects and a greater susceptibility to chronic disease. Though well-intentioned, these programs may ultimately have grave consequences for humanity.

SUSCEPTIBILITY IS INDIVIDUAL

As will be discussed in more depth in Chapter 5, one of the most important philosophical concepts in homeopathy is that disease and health must be analyzed and understood on an individual basis. Each person exists in a dynamically changing state that is unique to them. This state determines their most appropriate remedy as well as their individual susceptibility and reactivity to their environment.

Suppose that we have a man, woman, or child in a normal state of health. Along comes an *exciting cause* — a virus, bacteria, parasite, physical accident, emotional event, or stressful situation — that could potentially create a disturbance in their energetic and physical state. How will they react?

Partly, this depends on the strength and nature of the exciting cause. The stronger it is, the more likely that anyone, no matter who they are or what state they are in, will react to it in more or less the same way. For example, if someone hits their finger with a hammer, they will cry "ouch!" and develop a nasty bruise or broken finger. Their reaction will be quite predictable and less unique to them. For this reason, their treatment will also be more uniform, even within the homeopathic system; there will usually be a short list of commonly used homeopathic remedies for such situations. In the case of the hammer blow, the best remedy would most likely be *Arnica Montana* — a remedy derived from a mountain flower called leopard's bane. It is well known for its effectiveness in treating bruises, shock, and other kinds of physical trauma.

Another example of a strong exciting cause is a virulent epidemic. In such situations, most people develop similar symptoms, regardless of their individual constitution. For this reason, homeopathic treatment of epidemics is also less individualized. The homeopath's goal will be to find a small set of remedies that covers the symptoms that most people are experiencing — a set called the *genus epidemicus*. In a strong flu epidemic, for instance, the genus epidemicus will usually consist of two or three remedies that match the symptoms of that particular epidemic. Given such a small set of remedy choices, selecting the appropriate remedy for a particular patient is not very difficult. These remedies can also be used prophylactically if the threat of infection is imminent. Sandra Perko, PhD, has written an excellent book that discusses the success of homeopathy in the 1918 flu epidemic as well as potential remedies for future flu epidemics [Perko]. In my view, the information in this book would be far more effective and beneficial to the public than the yearly flu vaccination programs. Indeed, a brilliant aspect of homeopathy is that a genus epidemicus can be found for *any* epidemic — even of an unknown disease.

Since fairly uniform homeopathic treatment is possible in situations like trauma and epidemics, it is not surprising that conventional clinical trials of homeopathy have met with the greatest success in those situations that are also provoked by strong exciting causes and characterized by uniform patient responses. A good example is a study on the use of homeopathic remedies for severe pediatric diarrhea [Jacobs] that will be discussed at length in Chapter 7. It is only natural that a study constrained to using only a single predetermined remedy (or a small set of remedies) for a specific condition will be most successful when that condition can be characterized by predictable, not idiosyncratic, symptoms. In such situations, successful treatment is also much less dependent on the skill of the treating homeopath. Both of these factors make the outcome of conventionally designed trials more uniform and predictable.

But the forces that cause disease on a day-to-day basis are usually not as strong as a hammer blow nor as severe as an epidemic. In most situations, people will react differently to an exciting cause of disease, and their reaction will depend on their personal areas of weakness. Indeed, whether they react at all will depend on their susceptibility to the nature of the exciting cause. James Tyler Kent, MD, one of the most important American homeopaths of the late 1800s, wrote:

> "The one who is made sick is susceptible to the disease in accordance with the plane he is in and the degree of attenuation that happens to be present at the time of the contagion. The degree of the disease cause fits his susceptibility at the moment he is made sick." [Kent, p. 107]

In other words, there must be some kind of affinity between the disease cause and the state of the person who is susceptible to it. Another American homeopath of the early 1900s, Herbert A. Roberts, MD, wrote:

> "In analyzing susceptibility we find it is very largely an expression of a vacuum in the individual. The vacuum attracts and pulls for the things most needed, that are in the same plane of vibration as the want in the body... susceptibility has an attractive force which draws to itself the disease which is on the same plane of vibration and which tends to correct this... deficiency." [Roberts, p.151]

Roberts is implying here that the illnesses a person gets actually meet some kind of need within the person. Another way of thinking about this is in terms of a shaped hole (susceptibility) that is filled by a similarly shaped peg (disease). This type of reasoning, though certainly controversial, is worthy of some consideration. Many people feel that their disease experiences are also their teachers. Personally, I have found it quite instructive to consider *why* and *how* I get sick each time I do, and from more than just a physical point of view. What is the symbolism or meaning of a particular disease episode to the individual who experiences it?

For example, consider the modern scourge of lower back pain — or the more recent popular affliction, carpal tunnel syndrome. Why have these problems emerged in our society? Recent work in rehabilitative medicine by John Sarno, MD, links these types of conditions to emotional stress rather than to repetitive hand motions, bad seating choices, or hard physical labor [Sarno]. From a symbolic point of view, it makes sense that a person under severe work stress (unconsciously) develops the exact symptoms that will prevent them from continuing to perform their work — typing at a keyboard, sitting at a desk all day, or lifting heavy objects.

Rather than resorting to the normal diagnosis of slipped disc or repetitive stress injury and the resulting surgical treatment that goes along with it, Sarno has developed a "mind over pain" approach. The treatment simply consists of getting a patient to truly acknowledge and accept the actual root cause of their pain — stress. Sarno has found that this step alone can result in great therapeutic success and relief for a majority of his patients — even those who have suffered for many years and who manifest measurable signs of physical damage to their anatomy.

From a homeopathic point of view, Sarno's mind-cure requires patients to psychologically confront their emotional state head on, rather than suppress their feelings and hide behind a physical diagnosis. Indeed, Sarno has found that the surgical approach, which does not address the true root of the problem for many sufferers, is often unsuccessful in the long-term. I've used Sarno's technique myself. Several years ago, I myste- riously developed a case of "carpal tunnel syndrome." I had been typing at a computer terminal for 20 years without ill effect. Why were my wrists and hands aching and tingling now? After some thought, I realized that this condition developed after I had found out that my son Izaak would need surgery. I accepted the stress factor, and after his surgery, the pain completely left my hands and wrists.

CENTER OF GRAVITY

Another way of understanding individual susceptibility is to view each person's energetic state as having a *center of gravity* — a general zone of susceptibility to certain kinds of diseases. This notion was introduced by George Vithoulkas, a Greek homeopath who won the Right Livelihood Award in 1996, an alternative Nobel Prize conferred by the Swedish parliament. In his text, *The Science of Homeopathy* [Vithoulkas], Vithoulkas describes the center of gravity as a combination of states or vibratory levels in the emotional, mental, and physical realms. Within each of these realms is a range of diseases, from simple and largely benign, to serious and life-threatening.

Vithoulkas maintains that individuals resonate only with those diseases that have an affinity to their center of gravity. For example, a psychotic person's center of gravity is weighted very strongly in the mental and emotional realm, but not as strongly in the physical realm. This explains why psychotic patients do not get as many minor physical illnesses as other people. While they are very susceptible to stimuli that affect their minds, they are not as susceptible to factors that affect their bodies. In contrast, a cancer patient's center of gravity is very severe in the physical realm, but may be quite benign in the mental realm.

According to Vithoulkas's theory, a person tends to remain at the same center of gravity until they are shifted by some event to either a more severe level (by suppressive treatment or by some physical or emotional shock) or to a less severe level (by homeopathic treatment, for example). The center of gravity may also shift from one realm to another — for instance, from a primarily physical focus to a mental focus, or vice versa. Vithoulkas writes:

> "The principle of resonance renders the organism susceptible to influence on basically only one level at a given moment... Each level represents, for example, susceptibility to a particular range of diseases. If a person treated on Level B for gonorrhea receives antibiotics, his resonant frequency [may] change; over time, he will become susceptible to illnesses on, say, Level C. While experiencing symptoms of illness on this level, he will not acquire gonorrhea, even though he may be exposed... If however, such a person were to be treated homeopathically, the vibration rate would again move back down the scale, and the patient may well become susceptible to gonorrhea once again." [Vithoulkas, p. 82]

(Copyright © 1980 by George Vithoulkas. Used by permission of Grove/Atlantic, Inc.)

Assessing the movement of a patient's center of gravity is one way of determining whether they are getting better or are being suppressed by treatment. For example, it would be considered an excellent sign of improvement if a patient went from having chronic kidney infections to having minor skin problems, or from having schizophrenia to having severe allergies. But a progression from benign skin disease to severe depression would be a poor indicator — a sign that the center of gravity had been shifted in the wrong direction. Indeed, the grave side effects of many of today's "wonder drugs" are quite telling in this respect. For example, the acne medication Accutane is known to have the potential side effect of suicidal depression. Homeopathic philosophy clearly explains why this is so: because the suppression of acne shifts the center of gravity inward to more serious emotional disease.

Another interesting corollary of Vithoulkas's model is that it would be unlikely for a mentally and emotionally healthy person with minor physical ailments to suddenly and without cause develop a severe disease. Most people who become seriously ill have a history of increasingly poor physical or mental health, or they have experienced a severe jolt to their system — perhaps an extreme emotional or physical trauma or ill-advised drugging. Vithoulkas's model also implies that a lack of susceptibility to a particular ailment can be indicative of two things: that a person is *too healthy* to be affected or that they are *too sick* to be affected. Thus, just as a person who is healthy may not yield to the flu, a person who is very sick — for example, a psychotic patient — may not either. One might say that psychotic patients get sick less often. But the fact is, they are extremely sick all of the time, but in a different way.

History and Environment

What influences mold a person's state and create their unique susceptibility? One factor that both allopaths and homeopaths agree upon is basic physical constitution and inheritance. Each person is born with inherent weaknesses and proclivities. These are influenced by genetic makeup — inherited familial or racial tendencies. The susceptibilities of parents, and even of previous generations, are related to a person's current susceptibilities.

However, the homeopathic view of inherited susceptibility goes beyond genetics. For one thing, a person is viewed as inheriting not only genetic material from their parents, but also aspects of their vital forces. For this reason, many homeopaths believe that if an ancestor suffered from a serious disease (such as tuberculosis or venereal disease) or if their vital force was severely affected in some other way, a taint or effect from this experience may be transmitted to their descendants. For example, the descendants of a person who experienced tuberculosis might acquire the tendency to develop respiratory problems. Fortunately, homeopaths have also found that inherited disease tendencies can be cured homeo-pathically. Thus, even if a person's genes can't be altered, the proclivities of their vital force can be.

Curiously, research on the human genome has now revealed that the genetic code is far too simple to explain everything about us. Perhaps this provides further proof that it really is the vital force that is directing the show. Genes may only be receivers of information transmitted by the vital force, much like a television is only the receiver of a broadcast trans-mitted over the airwaves. Thus, just as fixing your television won't improve the quality of the shows you can receive on it, replacing or removing your body parts won't repair underlying problems with the vital force. And even if you can't replace your television (your genes), there is still the possibility of improving the quality of the programs it receives (the activity of the vital force).

Another factor that greatly influences a person's state and susceptibili-ty is their life history. What physical and emotional experiences have they had? What drugs, vaccinations, and other medicines have they taken? All of these factors help to shape the current state of a patient's mind, emotions, and body. If a person was repeatedly assaulted as a child, it will color the way they look at the world and the way they interact with others. Similarly, if a person has taken a great deal of drugs or has experienced severe phys-ical traumas, specific systems of their body will be left weakened.

From a homeopathic point of view, a person's life history also includes their gestation in the womb. Indeed, homeopaths have found that the experiences of a child's parents during conception and preg-nancy can provide invaluable information about the child. For example, it is not unusual for a pregnancy fraught with parental anxieties about work or money to result in a child that is chronically anxious and susceptible to anxiety-provoking situations, even if the parents themselves are not anxious by nature.

One illustrative case described by homeopath Julian Jonas, CCH, involved a child whose mother was abused by her spouse during pregnancy. The result was a child who was fearful, defensive, and violent. Ultimately, he was cured with a remedy that has the mental symptoms: *"Delusion: is being injured"* and *"Delusion: will receive injury."* The homeopath wrote, "What struck me as the clearest expression of his state was his statement that he feels people are trying to hurt him. This was the feeling that caused him to strike out to protect himself. It also probably reflects, to a certain extent, the mother's feeling during the first half of her pregnancy, while she was in the abusive relationship." [JJonas]

Another important factor that affects a person's susceptibility is their current living conditions and life habits. If a patient is living in rooms that are cold, damp, or unsanitary; is eating poorly; or is repeatedly exposed to chemicals via food or environment, their vitality will be weakened and their general susceptibility to disease will be greater. Indeed, their disease may simply be a direct result of these environmental factors. Homeopaths call these kinds of disease-provoking influences *maintaining causes*. Maintaining causes can be mental and emotional as well as physical — for example, a stressful job, an inappropriate school, or difficult family relations. Part of a homeopath's job is to inquire about such factors and to encourage patients, as much as possible, to remove maintaining causes from their lives.

As you can see, susceptibility is a complex thing, and understanding it is an important part of successful homeopathic treatment. A homeopath must consider the entire physical, emotional, and mental makeup of a patient and the full historical context of their case. From maintaining causes to exciting causes, from family inheritance to life history — all of these factors play roles in a patient's disease state. And when it comes to patient treatment and the quest for a true cure, the whole person must be addressed as well — a whole that is integrated, dynamic, and unique.

CHAPTER 5

⟨⟩

SYMPTOM PATTERNS: HUMANITY REFLECTED IN NATURE

"How can a plant or mineral contain within its nature, the similitude of a human psyche, a human ego, a human spirit? The fact that such a relationship does exist, and that this information is — somehow — within each separate species of plant, is a startling revelation, one that turns our understanding of life, biology, evolutionary theory and the nature of the manifest world itself on its proverbial ear... Shamans, seers and visionaries, both ancient and modern, have already voiced these connections for us. Still, all this might be idle speculation were it not for homeopathy itself. Homeopathic research or provings have given us the key to both prove and verify that such patterns of meaning exist... and have gone further to define the exact nature of this meaning. Homeopathy takes us out of the realm of subjectivity and overactive imagination and presents startling facts about how the natural realm mirrors our body and mind."

— Asa Hershoff, ND, DC, 2000 [Hershoff]

PSYCHOSOMATIC SYMPTOM PATTERNS

People often tease each other by saying, "Oh, that problem of yours is psychosomatic. It's all in your head." But there is actually truth to this statement. Homeopathy and all other holistic medical systems acknowledge that nearly every illness is "psychosomatic" — that is, incorporating aspects of both the psyche (mind) and soma (body). Moreover, each person manifests a psychosomatic pattern that is unique to them. It is the homeopath's job to discern this pattern and to match it to the symptom pattern of a remedy.

Of course, each remedy in the homeopathic materia medica has a distinctive psychosomatic pattern as well. This is true no matter what the remedy is made from — animal, plant, or mineral. The nature of a remedy's pattern is discovered by conducting a *proving* or remedy test. According to the Law of Similars, this remedy will be able to cure any patient whose pattern closely matches its own. Thus, in many ways, homeopathy is all about pattern discovery and pattern matching.

Jungian psychiatrist and homeopath Edward C. Whitmont, MD, wrote extensively in the area of psychosomatics. He felt that homeopathy was the only medical system that made a true science of this realm, and saw the homeopathic proving as an experimental method for determining the precise nature and range of human psychosomatic typology. In his book *Psyche and Substance* he wrote:

> "Our task would seem to lie in … finding the dynamic categories or laws which represent the common elements of … complementary psychic and physical evolutions. In short, we are looking for a 'generalized field theory' of psychosomatics. In order to avoid mere speculative theories, we must base our hypothesis upon observable or, still better, upon experimental material which would encompass psychic as well as somatic phenomena…The only such large-scale controlled psychosomatic experiments upon human beings are to be found in the so-called homeopathic 'provings.'" [Whitmont, pp. 14–15]

Whitmont actively researched the deeper meanings of psychosomatic remedy patterns and their relationship to the substances from which remedies are derived. Ultimately, he came to believe that a remedy's pattern reflects the underlying state of the originating substance. For example, the mental and physical symptoms elicited by a remedy made from animal matter can tell us something about the archetypal state of the animal itself, corresponding not only to its behavior and experience, but also to the mythology surrounding it. This fascinating area of study will be discussed at the end of this chapter. For now, let's begin by taking a look at some psychosomatic patterns.

ARNICA — THE TRAUMA REMEDY

As mentioned in the previous chapter, one of the most commonly used remedies in the homeopathic medicine chest is *Arnica Montana* — a remedy made from a little yellow mountain flower called leopard's bane. Arnica is usually one of the first remedies to be considered in cases of trauma and shock. Indeed, it is sometimes called the "fall herb," because it is so commonly needed after a nasty fall. If your child has just tumbled out of a tree, or you've just bumped your head and feel bruised and disoriented, consider Arnica. Indeed, any situation in which the body feels sore and discombobulated may be a call for this remedy. For instance, it is a favorite for postoperative shock and soreness, jet lag, and for use after a dentist's appointment, when the jaw feels sore and the nerves feel rattled. Allopathic surgeons have also been known to use Arnica; a prominent Manhattan plastic surgeon once confessed to me that he uses it postoperatively for many of his patients. Of course, this remedy should only be used when a patient's symptoms actually match those of Arnica.

Mentally, the Arnica state is characterized by either a dazed, numbed-out apathy, or by fearful anxiety — a common polarity found in shock cases. Sometimes, the patient may say that they are "just fine," even if this is clearly not the case. They may even answer questions correctly, despite the fact that they are nearly unconscious. On the other hand, they may be shouting and delirious. The typical Arnica patient also wants to be left alone; in fact, they may fear being approached or touched. Just think about how you feel after you've just fallen off a bicycle or walked into a wall, and you might get the idea. The Arnica symptom pattern also includes dizziness that occurs upon closing one's eyes — a symptom commonly found in such situations.

A textbook case of Arnica once presented itself to me on a school field trip. A child in my son's class fell and bumped his head. He just sat there in a dazed stupor, even after several minutes had passed. Although he said he was fine, something was clearly amiss. After discussing the situation with some other parents and the child, I gave him a single dose of Arnica. Much to everyone's amazement and my delight, he was up again within a minute, running about and getting into lots of trouble once more.

In the materia medica compiled by Indian homeopath Dr. S. R. Phatak (a compact materia medica that is a favorite among practitioners), the mental symptoms of Arnica are described as follows:

"MIND: *Fear*, of being struck or touched; or approached; of sickness; of instant death; with cardiac distress at night; of space; on awakening; of crowd, public places. Morose, repentant mood. Mentally prostrate and apathetic, but physically restless; says nothing ails him. When spoken to, answers slowly with effort. Feels well in serious cases. Forgetful, what he reads, quickly escapes his mind. After rage sheds tears and makes exclamations. Hopeless; indifferent. Violent attacks of anguish... A sudden fear that rouses one from sleep at night, especially after an accident. Coma. Muttering delirium. Sensation of being good for nothing. Easily frightened, unexpected trifles cause him to start. Sits as if in thought." [Phatak, p. 66]

Of course, an Arnica patient need not exhibit all of these symptoms. What is important is that their symptoms be included within the remedy's larger pattern of symptoms and that the two patterns match overall. Phatak's description of the Arnica mental state also illustrates the kinds of symptoms that are associated with remedies in general. Nearly every remedy has a unique mental pattern of this kind.

Naturally, Arnica has many physical symptoms too. The materia medica for this remedy (and for most remedies) includes detailed symptoms for all areas of the body, including: head, eyes, ears, nose, face, mouth, stomach, abdomen, urinary tract, genitals (including sexual behavior), respiratory system, heart, neck and back, extremities, skin, and fever-related symptoms. Another important aspect of a remedy symptom pattern is its *modalities* — general conditions or situations that improve or aggravate symptoms. For instance, symptoms may improve or become aggravated in certain types of weather, at certain times of the day, or from eating particular foods.

Because remedy patterns are so vast in scope, committing them to memory can be a formidable task. One helpful strategy is to try to find a theme that links all of the symptoms of a remedy together. In the case of Arnica, this theme or thread of meaning is *trauma*. Thus, not only is Arnica a potential remedy in actual cases of trauma, but it is also a likely remedy when a patient's symptoms resemble a traumalike state.

For example, one trauma-related theme that runs through many of Arnica's physical symptoms is *blood*. These blood-related symptoms include: bloodshot eyes; redness of the cheeks and throat; a tendency to hemorrhage or bleed (from the retina, ears, nose, or the uterus after sex); bruising in general; vomiting of blood; bloody stools; and profuse menstruation. Arnica's modalities also reflect a traumatized state. A person who will benefit from this remedy is generally aggravated by touch, motion, damp coldness, mental or physical shocks, and from lying on the left side (because of heart symptoms). Their sleep will tend to be restless and punctuated by night terrors. On the flip side, Arnica patients generally feel better from clear, cold, stimulating weather and from lying down with the head in a lowered position — not a surprising modality for actual trauma states, but it also holds true in other situations calling for Arnica.

Given all the accidents that can occur in everyday life, the Arnica pattern is clearly a commonly occurring one. Nearly anyone who uses homeopathy has their own amazing Arnica stories to tell. Here's a typical anecdote from homeopath Will Taylor, MD:

> "Three years ago my sons were tearing around the house, and Caleb slammed the dining room door while Ben had his hand in the jam (the hinge side). There was a horrible crunching sound and I opened the door to see his hand with three fingers fractured and deviated... I took advantage of that 'Arnica moment' between injury and full consciousness and set his fingers by distraction, and gave him a 1M [dose] of Arnica. The next couple of days he tended to protect the hand... a bit, but used it for Legos now and then without complaint, and there was only some minimal purpura [bruising]. That was it. I have no idea why

we might need a double-blind trial. If I could do that with placebo, I'd be wicked pleased." [WT3]

Note that a "1M dose of Arnica" means that a tincture of the Arnica flower was repeatedly diluted in a ratio of 1:100 (1 drop combined with 99 drops of water) 1,000 times. That means that the Arnica flower was diluted to a ratio of $1:10^{2,000}$ — that's 1 followed by 2,000 zeros! Avogadro's number — the point at which a molecule of substance would no longer likely be present — is merely 10^{23}. Here is another Arnica story:

> "I had a case of a little boy who fell on his face and severely loosened one of his front teeth. It remained loose and began to darken. The dentist wanted to remove it. The parents called me, and I suggested Arnica. Not only did the gum tighten around the tooth in very short order so that it was no longer loose, but also all discoloration in the tooth faded, and it is now white and beautiful, and appears totally healthy." [VCD]

The next Arnica anecdote, which describes the experiences of a student attending a course on homeopathy, illustrates the wide-reaching effects that a remedy can have.

> "One of the main things that I took home with me the first day is to minimize use of drugs that suppress the body's own healing process. That evening, I strained my knee. I'd had off-and-on knee pain for a year. It really hurt and scared me. Instead of heading for the anti-inflammatory medicine, I used Arnica Montana... During the second day... Dr. Shevin was talking about his own case of poison ivy. He had tried the typical homeopathic remedies without success. During his explanation he demonstrated his computer program's search capabilities for homeopathic remedies. His main sensation was that of 'soreness.' The search yielded the remedy Arnica. As he was describing this, I thought about how I itched this morning from the rash on my neck that the dermatologist had diagnosed as eczema the day before class started. I reached up to feel for it. It was *gone!* My mouth dropped open in amazement. Since the class, my knee has stayed painless and the rash has not returned. What could be better than that? Homeopathy works." [Evans]

Of course, I have Arnica stories of my own to tell, and some are less typical. It turns out that Max's mental clarity and ability to communicate was often helped somewhat by Arnica. I noticed this early on, even when he was taking his daily doses of Carcinosin, because we would usually give him some Arnica after dental appointments. Of course, Max's response to Arnica also made sense, since Arnica is homeopathic to a dazed and unconscious sort of state, which is also characteristic of autism.

Arnica also came in handy for Max in a mild case of whooping cough. We tried a few common whooping cough remedies, but they only had a temporary effect on him. Finally, I noticed that his eyes had become bloodshot from all the coughing. I could find only two remedies listed for this particular symptom (bloodshot eyes from coughing), and one of them was Arnica. It also just happened to be a minor whooping cough remedy. A dose or two of Arnica ended the whooping cough completely.

By this point, you should have some feeling for the Arnica state and how it manifests itself as a cohesive psychosomatic pattern. Personally, I wouldn't go anywhere without this remedy; I always carry some in my purse, just in case. But despite the fact that Arnica can be truly wonderful in most trauma situations, it isn't *always* the answer. The patterns have to match up. And this homeopathic pattern matching game — matching remedy pattern to patient pattern — becomes even more difficult when patient responses to disease are more individualized.

For example, consider the treatment of coughs. There are hundreds of ways that a cough can present itself if you truly examine its precise characteristics. Indeed, almost every remedy in the materia medica has its own unique cough symptoms. How to choose the best one for a particular case of cough? There are really two answers to this question. One involves the mechanics of homeopathic practice — the techniques that homeopaths use to select a remedy. The second involves the art of homeopathy — the ability to understand the nature and meaning of a patient's pattern and find its analogue in a remedy. We will now consider each of these important aspects of homeopathic prescribing in more detail.

The Mechanics of Matching Symptom Patterns

When my family first started using homeopathy, our homeopath told us that it was a much more complex system of medicine than allopathy. I didn't really believe him at the time, but now I do. It is easy to get lost in the myriad symptoms of patients and remedies; matching patient patterns to remedy patterns can often be elusive. Long-term case management can be even more difficult.

Of course, homeopaths have come up with a variety of strategies and tools for effective practice. First and foremost, a homeopath must master the art of *case-taking* — i.e., gathering information during a patient interview. He or she must also become an astute observer of patient appearance and behavior. Don't forget: without high-quality information about a patient, a homeopath will have a hard time finding their matching remedy. For this reason, an important part of homeopathic training is learning how to elicit as much reliable psychological and physical information as possible. Homeopaths also learn how to distinguish between a patient's true inner state and the superficial mask they may hide behind.

After case information has been gathered, a homeopath's next task is to select a patient's most important and useful symptoms — the symptoms that will most likely guide them to the curative remedy. This step alone can take years to master. It requires insight (for instance, recognizing that a particular symptom might be symbolic of a larger portion of the patient's overall case) and experience with the materia medica (knowing that certain symptoms are more likely to lead to fruitful remedies than others). In fact, it is not unusual for a master homeopath to select only three or four symptoms to analyze. In contrast, a novice homeopath may sit with dozens of symptoms and not quite know how to make sense of them.

Finally, the homeopath must analyze the chosen symptoms and make a final remedy determination. Naturally, experienced homeopaths know a great deal of materia medica by heart and will have a good idea of which remedies to consider right after the patient interview. But even if they have vast experience, no homeopath can memorize the entire materia medica, which encompasses thousands of pages of remedy descriptions. At best, they can maintain solid familiarity with a hundred or so commonly used remedies. While one of these remedies may be able to provide relief to most patients, it is not unusual for a more obscure remedy to be the simillimum.

To cope with this problem, homeopaths have devised a reference tool that enables quick access to all of the remedies associated with a particular symptom — a *repertory*. A repertory contains a listing of symptoms, organized in a methodical and logical fashion. Each of these symptoms is then followed by the list of remedies associated with that symptom. This symptom/remedy-list pairing is called a *rubric*. For example, in the "Cough" chapter of Kent's repertory (compiled by turn-of-the-20th-century American homeopath James Tyler Kent, MD [KentRep]), a homeopath can look up the rubric for whooping cough and find the names of 118 remedies. Many of the rubrics in homeopathic repertories are amazingly specific. For example, in the "Hearing" section of Kent's repertory we have the rubric:

"Hearing: Impaired, before a storm: Nux-m."

In other words, the remedy *Nux Moschata* (made from nutmeg) is associated with hearing impairment that occurs before a storm. This rubric illustrates how odd rubrics can be. Interestingly, it is unusual symptoms like this one that can lead directly to a remedy choice for a patient.

Using repertories, homeopaths can look up thousands of symptoms, ranging from common cold symptoms to ones as obscure as the nutmeg symptom above, and they can get ideas about potential remedies for their patients. By looking up several symptoms at once and intersecting the sets of remedies associated with them, the prospective remedies for a patient can be narrowed down further. In the days before computers, homeopaths used special "repertorizing sheets" to perform this task manually. Today, computerized repertory programs enable homeopaths to quickly perform complex analyses that would have taken hours in the past. Once this repertorization process is complete and the set of likely remedies has been sufficiently narrowed, a homeopath will finalize his or her analysis by reading the materia medica descriptions of the top contending remedies. They will then select the one that seems the most suitable overall.

Now, this may all sound simple in concept. But in truth, even with today's computerized repertory programs, one can easily get lost. What if the chosen symptoms are so common that each is associated with hundreds of remedies, and intersecting them gets you no closer? What if you pick an extraneous symptom that really isn't that important and it unnecessarily limits your view of the possible remedy choices? Invariably, repertorization is only a means toward an end for the homeopath. The real problem lies in knowing what's important in a patient's case in the first place. It's knowing how to look at a patient's life story and recognize where the golden thread lies — the center of the case, the meaning that underlies a patient's unique symptom pattern.

THE CENTER OF THE CASE

In the last chapter we discussed the holistic nature of disease — how disease is a body-mind phenomenon, not just a pile of isolated physical symptoms. Because disease is a state of the whole person, the most significant and fruitful symptoms will be those that tell us something about the whole person as well, not just about a particular part of their body. For example, consider the symptom: "My elbow is sore." This symptom would not be very helpful in finding a remedy because it says nothing about the person as a whole. But a symptom like "When it rains, I get sore joints and feel depressed" is much more useful. It may even lead directly to the simillimum, because it says something about the entire body and mind and how it responds to a particular condition.

Why are general, holistic symptoms so important and useful? Remember that the true root of a person's disease lies in a disturbance to their vital force. As a result, the most fruitful therapeutic strategy will be to cure this root, this central disturbance in the patient's energetic state, rather than its various outward physical manifestations. Dr. Rajan Sankaran, an Indian homeopath, writes:

> "The central disturbance... comes first and this is followed by changes
> in the various organ systems depending upon each individual's patho-

logical tendencies. Pathology grows on the central disturbance like a creeper on a stick. What we have to do is remove the central disturbance." [Sankaran, p. 6]

So how can we discover this central disturbance? The answer is to search for those symptoms that most characterize it. Usually, these will be the symptoms that the person identifies with as part of their whole being; for instance, the symptom "I get depressed when it rains." Homeopaths call these *general symptoms*. In contrast, *particular symptoms* are those symptoms that pertain to a particular part of the body — "My elbow is sore."

There are many kinds of general symptoms. For example, the tendency to be hot or cold; to have a certain sweating pattern, sleep pattern, or sexual proclivity; and to have certain intense food cravings and aversions are all examples of general symptoms. Notice that when describing any of these symptoms, a patient will usually use the word "I": "I sweat on my chest at night," "I can't sleep between 3 A.M. and 4 A.M." "I hate sex," "I love spicy food and I absolutely hate fish." In contrast, when describing a *particular* symptom, the word "my" is used: "My knee hurts," "My eyes are itchy." However, when several particular symptoms form a repeating pattern, they begin to take on the characteristics of a more general symptom. Thus, "My elbow is sore" and "My knee is sore" and "My wrist is sore" start looking like the more general symptom "I have sore joints."

Many general symptoms can be directly observed by a homeopath. For instance, is a patient thin or flabby, dry or sweaty, nervous or calm, quick or slow moving? General characteristics like these are important in all holistic medicines because they say something about a person's overall physical and emotional nature.

Of course, some symptoms are more important than others. Intense and frequently experienced symptoms are given more weight than fleeting or less–reliable ones. Homeopaths also tend to give greater weight to subjectively experienced symptoms. Thus, it is more useful to know that a patient feels hot, along with details that describe the experience of heat — its sensation, what makes it better or worse, etc. — than to simply know a patient's thermometer reading. Subjective symptoms also tend to be "I" symptoms; they relate to how a person feels within themself. For example, "I feel very hot and clammy when I'm about to meet new people." In contrast, a temperature-reading is a particular symptom, because it measures only a particular feature of the body — "My temperature is 100 degrees."

Perhaps the most important of the "I" symptoms are mental and emotional symptoms. After all, they lie closest to the core of a person. Indeed, if mental and emotional symptoms are highly pronounced and characteristic of a person, it is not unusual for a homeopathic prescription to be based primarily on them. Such a prescription can even cure physical pathology that is not otherwise associated with the prescribed remedy. A typical case that illustrates this point was related by Dr. Sankaran.

> "A case of severe cough in a boy taught me much about the importance of mental symptoms. The cough would not subside even after several remedies were tried. The parents were getting anxious. The child was restless, very stubborn and did the very opposite of what he was told to do. On the basis that *Tuberculinum* is a good remedy for persistent respiratory complaints, restlessness and obstinacy, it was given but did not work. One day when the boy was sitting in my clinic, suddenly he did something very funny. He shouted at me, 'Hey, Sankaran, your medicines are useless; better give me some good medicine, else I will not come here.' This, coming from a boy of five, uttered in a violent, threatening tone was shocking. I gathered from the parents that his behaviour at home was funny. He was disobedient, shrieking, mocking, quarrelsome. He was intensely restless. He threw things or destroyed them. However, he reacted to music favourably, would dance to tunes. I was not accustomed to think of *Tarentula* [a remedy associated with these behavioral symptoms] for cough. Maybe, I thought, when Tarentula covers the mind so well, it may cover the rest of the symptoms too. The response to Tarentula was magical in two days, whereas I had struggled over it for weeks with other remedies, and failed. Even his behaviour improved." [Sankaran, p. 82]

This case illustrates the importance of prioritizing symptoms when choosing a remedy. After many failed attempts to cure this boy's cough with cough remedies, Sankaran decided to focus more on the boy's striking and perhaps even more problematic mental and emotional symptoms. This case also demonstrates that an important criterion for prioritizing symptoms is their peculiarity. In this instance, it was the boy's behavior that was most peculiar, not his cough. If homeopathic prescribing can be likened to solving a mystery, with symptoms as the clues, the words of Sherlock Holmes are most apt: *"That which is out of the common is usually a guide rather than a hindrance... That which seemingly confuses the case is the very thing that furnishes the clue to its solution."*

Homeopaths call a truly unusual symptom a *"strange, rare, or peculiar"* (SRP). Mental, emotional, behavioral, or physical SRPs (for example, the unusual hearing symptom of nutmeg) can be remarkably helpful in homeopathic prescribing, not only because fewer remedies are associated with them, but because such symptoms tend to more closely represent or symbolize the central disturbance of a case. If nearly everyone experiences an ailment in the same way, its symptoms won't be very revealing about a patient as an individual. But if a symptom is very unusual and striking, it says something interesting and unique about the patient — and it is often symbolic of their inner state.

Consider, for example, the symptom: *"Delusion, that he walks on his knees."* This odd symptom is associated with the remedy *Baryta Carbonica* (made from carbonate of barium), a remedy that is also associated with strong feelings of inferiority. The Baryta Carbonica patient's delusion that he is walking on his knees is most likely symbolic of his inner feelings of inferiority.

Physical SRP symptoms can provide invaluable insight into a case as well. Consider, for example, the following symptom from Kent's repertory [KentRep]:

"Eye: Moonlight ameliorates: Aurum."

In other words, if a patient has the unusual experience that their eye symptoms are ameliorated by moonlight, they may also be a candidate for the remedy *Aurum* — made from potentized gold. Now, why would an Aurum patient's eye symptoms be ameliorated in this way? What is the meaning of this symptom? How does it fit into the Aurum symptom pattern?

Aurum patients tend to set high standards for themselves. They are also inclined to be overly responsible, prideful, and guilt-laden. They can even become suicidal if they do not meet their self-imposed goals and responsibilities. Just like a king who wears the golden crown, Aurum, made from potentized gold, tries to bear the full burden of his or her kingdom and would rather die than fail.

Interestingly, in most cultures, gold is also symbolically linked with the sun. And, as it turns out, the sun is associated mythologically with many of the symptoms of Aurum. Whitmont writes:

> "Astrologically, the solar [sun] principle stands for the life will in the individualizing human consciousness, the sense of self-value, honesty, responsibility, pride, willpower, vital strength and the capacity to exert control, all vested in the heart." [Whitmont, p. 158]

Aurum is a well-known remedy for heart problems. It also has an affinity to the eyes, the receivers of the sun's light. Given the intense responsibilities and self-expectations that Aurum patients tend to take upon themselves, perhaps it makes sense that their eye symptoms are ameliorated by the lesser and perhaps more comforting light of the moon — the sun's less demanding sister.

Now, I know that this will sound like a stretch to most readers. "You mean, the mythology associated with gold or the sun has something to do with Aurum's symptoms?" Well, yes! But the real point is, these correspondences are not merely speculative — *they have been borne out by remedy provings.* The homeopathic use of Aurum for heart or eye symptoms is *not* based on mythological speculations about gold or the sun — it is based on the symptoms that have arisen during provings of Aurum. Nevertheless, these mythological connections do exist, and they certainly make for fascinating and illuminating study. As I will discuss later on in this chapter, they may also provide insight into deeper phenomena that may be going on in the world that surrounds us.

MODALITIES AND CONCOMITANTS

If unusual symptoms are so useful, how can we find more of them? One strategy is to gather more and more information about a symptom until it becomes unusual or characteristic in some way. For example, we can try to identify the precise location and sensation of a symptom, the way it tends to begin and end, and the speed at which it develops: "The pain is like the sting of a needle in my left shoulder. It comes on suddenly, and then shoots down to my left elbow."

Another fruitful strategy is to collect symptom *modalities*. As described earlier, a modality is something that aggravates or ameliorates a symptom; for example, the person whose joints are sore when it rains. There are many kinds of modalities. Symptoms may become worse or better at certain times of the day or in certain locales like the mountains or seaside. They may also be affected by specific seasons and types of weather, phases of the menstrual cycle, physical positions or motions, or emotional or other kinds of situations.

Another feature that can provide distinctiveness to a symptom are its *concomitants* — coexisting symptoms that, on the face of things, seem unrelated to the symptom in question but somehow always occur at the same time. It is this coupling of symptoms that makes them unusual and distinctive. Concomitants may link physical and emotional symptoms (for instance, indigestion and depression) or seemingly unrelated physical symptoms (vertigo and thirst).

The treatment of simple coughs provides an excellent illustration of the importance of symptom modalities and concomitants. There are hundreds of cough remedies, with at least 20 that are commonly used. Each one of them has its own unique cough characteristics. Table 1 provides just a few examples (derived from [Castro, Panos]). It will give you a feeling for the kinds of information that are needed to fully individualize a symptom and may also give you an idea of how difficult homeopathic prescribing can be, even for a simple cough. And yet, with the right remedy, a cough can be quickly and completely cured — not simply palliated or suppressed.

Table 1: Characteristics of Four Common Cough Remedies

Aconitum Napellus
(Monkshood flower)

- Cough after exposure to cold, dry wind.
- Sudden onset.
- Constant, short, dry, croupy.
- Wakes in night with cough, feels anxious and fearful.
- Worse in the evening and night, in a warm room, or from dry cold wind.
- Better from open air.
- Important for the first stage of croup.

Antimonium Tartaricum
(Tartrate of Antimony and Potash, mineral)

- A persistent cough with a rattling chest; can't spit up mucus.
- Feels cold and sweaty with a pale face.
- Weak, drowsy, gasps for breath.
- Worse in the evening, from lying down, from warmth, from damp cold weather, from sour foods and liquids, and from milk.
- Better from sitting up, in a cold open room, from expectoration.

Phosphorus
(The element)

- Hard, dry, tickling, exhausting cough, with trembling.
- "Clergyman's Sore Throat"; violent tickling while speaking.
- Sensation of heaviness, weight on chest.
- Feels cold, weak, anxious, hoarse, sweats at night.
- Worse in the evening, from inhaling cold air, laughing, talking, touch, warm food or drink, change of weather, getting wet in hot weather.
- Better in open air, after sleep, from cold food.
- Thirsty for ice cold drinks.

Pulsatilla
(Windflower)

- Loose in morning, with thick yellow mucus; dry at night.
- Coughing fits with gagging or choking.
- Cough disturbs sleep.
- Thirstless, with dry mouth.
- Weepy, wants sympathy, clingy, changeable mood.
- Craves fresh air, which ameliorates. Also better from moving around and from cold applications.
- Worse from warm room, in the evening, from lying down, or from becoming overheated.

CAUSATION

Another aspect of a symptom that can make it more characteristic (indeed, perhaps its most important feature if it's available) is its *causation* — the physical or emotional event that seemed to have triggered or preceded it. In my own experience, simply reflecting on what happened just before a symptom appeared can sometimes get rid of it. The next time you get a cough or headache, think about what happened just before it began — perhaps an upsetting or aggravating event. If you process this information rather than suppress it, it is often enough to remove the physical symptom entirely. The following story from my own experience underscores the importance of causation in homeopathic prescribing.

Several years ago I received a very disturbing phone call from my schizophrenic brother. Right afterward, I developed a short tickling cough. Just an hour later, I seemed to be really coming down with something. Soon, I developed a fever and was feeling quite sick. I called my homeopath, and he recommended a low dose of *Aconite*, a remedy that can quickly nip colds and coughs in the bud, especially if they come on quickly and if the remedy is given right at the onset. Somehow, though, I had forgotten to tell him about the phone call from my brother; it had slipped my mind.

The Aconite helped quite a bit that evening, but the next day, everything got worse again. I developed a high fever and was completely prostrate. Rather than redosing with Aconite again, my homeopath decided to switch me to a new remedy. Over the course of the next few weeks, the remedies he recommended helped somewhat, but they never cured what eventually turned into a persistent bronchitis. Each night, I would cough and cough, and the remedies only palliated.

After a month of this, I began to reflect more about the whole episode. Suddenly, I remembered how it all began — with that phone call from my brother. I called the homeopath, and he suggested that I try Aconite again — this time in a much higher dose. By the next morning, my bronchitis and cough were completely gone. Why?

Besides being an excellent remedy for the early stages of acute coughs and colds, Aconite is also one of the most important remedies for ailments resulting from fear. Remember, Aconite had helped me considerably that first night. But the single low dose I had taken was not enough to cure me. If my homeopath had been aware of the causative event for my cough, he would probably have followed that initial dose with another — because Aconite embodied the state that led to my illness. As Phatak writes in his materia medica,

"The rapidity of action of Aconite determines its symptomatology. Its symptoms are *acute, violent, and painful.* They appear *suddenly...* Mind is affected by such emotional factors as *fright, shock, vexation.* Nerves are excited and the patient remains under emotional and nervous tension... Great anxiety. *Agonizing fear and restlessness* accompany every ailment however trivial." [Phatak, pp. 5–6]

My main reaction to my brother's call had been fear. And just as Aconite causes quick and dramatic physical effects, often in reaction to fear, my reaction to my brother's phone call immediately triggered a cough that quickly developed into bronchitis. I was in an Aconite state. Even after I had erroneously taken other remedies for my cough, I was still in an Aconite state, weeks later. For this reason, another high dose of Aconite terminated the whole affair. Afterward, I began to feel stronger and less fearful about my interactions with my brother as well.

SITUATION

One of the reasons why a causative event can be the key to finding a curative remedy is that, quite frequently, this event says something about the nature of a person's central disturbance. Perhaps the causation is a traumatic physical accident, an acute illness, an upsetting emotional event, or exposure to a toxic chemical or drug. All of these things can dramatically alter a person's state. Often, a patient will report that they have never been quite the same since that time. In cases like this, the triggering event has actually caused the patient's energetic state to become frozen. They have assumed a psychophysical "stance" or response in order to deal with the event, but they have remained in that stance long after the event has passed. As a result, they now see the world through a lens that doesn't quite fit anymore. Eventually, their psyche and body will become distorted by this unsuitable posture, and the net effect will be disease.

Indian homeopath Rajan Sankaran calls this frozen or erroneous stance toward life a person's *situation*. In his books *The Spirit of Homoeopathy* [Sankaran] and *The Soul of Remedies* [Sankaran97], he describes the situation of many remedies in the materia medica. For example, a person who needs *Kali Bromatum* (potassium bromide) acts like a person who "has to be extremely vigilant not to do anything wrong. It is as if his survival depends on it; as if he will be cast away if something goes wrong... As a child... in a family where the parents are very strict morally." [Sankaran, p. 284]

Now, a person need not have had such a childhood to assume a Kali Bromatum stance towards life. But something must have happened that caused them to feel this way. As a result, they develop the characteristic pattern of Kali Bromatum. This pattern includes an anxious restlessness (especially restless, fidgety hands and a tendency to constantly look around); suspiciousness; a fear of people; and the feeling that something terrible is going to happen. Mentally, a Kali Bromatum patient may be foggy, with memory loss and trouble speaking or writing. They will also tend to feel guilty — as if they have committed a crime or are about to commit one.

The physical symptoms of Kali Bromatum also mirror its tense, anxious, and guilty mental nature. These symptoms include many neurological problems — paralysis; epilepsy; spasticity (for example, spastic colon, persistent hiccough, and stammering); and feelings of numbness. Just reading these symptoms creates a vivid image of this kind of person, doesn't it? Indeed, these symptoms form a coherent pattern of meaning — a pattern that can be understood as an underlying situational stance toward life. If a homeopath can tease a situation like this out of the many mental and physical symptoms reported by a patient, and then match it to a remedy, they will be very close to finding the patient's simillimum.

THE DOCTRINE OF SIGNATURES

It is truly amazing that the totality of symptoms caused (and cured) by a highly diluted substance can actually take the form of a coherent pattern. Who would imagine that ingesting some incredibly dilute and potentized potassium bromide could cause such related mental and physical phenomena? Somehow, the potentization process seems to be able to bring out strong characteristic effects from even the most mundane and otherwise benign substances — for instance, *Natrum Muriaticum* is an important and powerful remedy made from ordinary salt.

What is even more amazing, however, is that the pattern caused by a potentized remedy can be symbolically related to the material substance from which it was derived. This can be seen most easily with animal remedies. The mental and physical symptoms of such remedies are nearly always related to the behavior or mythology associated with the animal from which they were made. But the same is true for plant and mineral remedies too. The environment and climate in which a plant grows best, the soil nutrients it prefers, its relationship to other plants, its physical shape, and especially the mythology surrounding it — all of these factors are usually related to the mental and physical symptoms associated with a plant remedy. Mineral remedy symptoms can also be related to where the mineral is found, what it is typically used for, and the myths associated with it.

This phenomenon — the relationship between a remedy's symptoms and its source material — is called the *doctrine of signatures*. In medieval times, the doctrine of signatures was understood and used in a fairly superficial way. For example, the heartlike shape of a flower was taken as a sign that it might be useful for heart ailments. Today, however, many homeopath's view the doctrine of signatures as a much deeper phenomenon. It seems to imply that the universe is inherently symbolic; that somehow, inherent patterns of meaning are embedded within us and within every plant, animal, and mineral — patterns that can have causal effects upon one another. Moreover, this phenomenon is not merely speculative. It has been repeatedly borne out by blind provings

(provings in which the source substance was not revealed) and by the Law of Similars itself. While homeopathic doctrine clearly dictates that this phenomenon not be used as a basis for treatment (treatment must be based on proving data), many homeopaths do use this kind of information as an intuitive aid for understanding remedies and their patterns.

Consider this. If the doctrine of signatures really holds true — if the archetypal meaning of a substance is somehow embedded physically within it and is released by the process of potentization — it may enable us to understand the universe in a whole new way. To discover the inherent meaning hidden within any plant, animal, or mineral, we need only potentize it and test it in a proving. The proving process might be an entryway into unbelievable knowledge.

While it may seem like a mere trick of the imagination to many people, on some level, I believe that the doctrine of signatures also makes sense. After all, humans are biological organisms that evolved within the web of meaning of this world. Perhaps it is no accident that, mirrored within some other substance within that web, is our own counterpart — a substance whose very essence mirrors our own distortions and diseased state. For example, is it really a coincidence that a woman who was later cured by *Lac Felinum* (cat's milk) also happened to be so "catlike" that her friends called her "a cat"? If such a person manifested physical symptoms that were caused in a blind proving of cat's milk, is it any wonder that she seemed catlike to the people who knew her?

Whitmont had much to say about this phenomenon in his book, *Psyche and Substance*. For example, in the following, he relates it to alchemy:

> "Medieval alchemists held man to be a microcosmic replica of the macrocosmos of nature... This contention is experimentally and clinically borne out by Homeopathy. Every disturbance of health, be it organic or merely functional, is... a cry for the process that is its macrocosmic form analogon and that can restore balance when brought into confrontation with the disease process." [Whitmont, p. xiii]

Whitmont also tried to relate the doctrine of signatures to Carl Jung's notion of synchronicity. Jung believed that external events can have inherent meaning that correspond synchronistically to inner psychic events. For example, he believed that it was no accident that a clock would stop ticking the instant its owner died. Whitmont similarly speculated that it was no accident that a person's disease pattern reflects the symbolism associated with the substance that will cure them. He wrote:

> "When one's course of life passes through a 'field of meaning,' this field manifests itself through events on various levels (for instance, psyche and soma), all of them in their own different fashion giving expression to that same formative factor." [Whitmont, p. 85]

Thus, the Aconite flower and the fear-related ailments it can cure are both parts of the same field of meaning — a field into which a person enters after experiencing a frightening event.

Whitmont also believed that the Law of Similars was a general principle, applicable to all analogous or synchronistic phenomena, even beyond the realm of healing. He wrote, "*The law of similars is the law of the basic relationship of analogous phenomena.*" [Whitmont, p. 32] What if this is true? What other discoveries might be made if the Law of Similars were applied to other purposes besides medicinal ones? What exactly is going on in the energetic realm when we bring two similar fields of meaning together?

ANIMAL PATTERNS

There are many homeopaths who shy away from discussion of the doctrine of signatures. Certainly, the concept is controversial, and it is not necessary for effective homeopathic practice. But it *is* fascinating. Consider, for example, how it manifests itself in animal remedies. One of the most striking new remedies is *Androctonus*. Derived from scorpion poison (but, of course, administered in dilute nonmaterial doses), Androctonus was proved in 1985 on 31 volunteers. The proving was blind — both the provers and the supervisors who recorded their symptoms did not know what substance they were testing — but it still yielded the following emotional symptoms [Vermeulen]:

- A heightened feeling of overconfidence.
- Contemptuousness and defiance.
- A lacking in moral feeling.
- Quarrelsomeness.
- Unsympathetic feeling. Cruel and unfeeling.
- Deceitfulness.
- A delusion that one is about to be assaulted.
- A malicious desire to injure others.
- Suspiciousness.
- A lack of control over one's impulses.
- Indifference to pleasure or to one's surroundings or to other people's welfare or opinions.
- Anxiety and fear, ameliorated from walking around.
- Aversion to company, with a feeling that one is alone or separated from the world.
- Emotions that are easily excited.

Notice how evocative many of these symptoms are of the impressions most people have about scorpions — violent, cruel, and antisocial. Indeed, scorpions are generally loners that are so aggressive that they will eat one another. When hunting, they usually let their prey come to them, and they can accurately detect a potential victim's location by sensing the vibrations caused by their movements. These characteristics are echoed in the case described below. A truck driver who was later cured with Androctonus describes his passion for hunting:

> "Nothing stops me from doing what I want to do. I spent a lot of my early years alone. I entertained myself... As a child, my father was away at war. We used to play soldiers and I was better at it than the other kids. I was the only kid on the block with a bow and arrow and a tomahawk... Two brothers — I kicked their butts... As a child I spent a lot of time with my grandmother. She was part American Indian... I learned about being in tune with nature, about animals. I learned how to manipulate situations... Killing is not a sport. I'm dead serious about it. I know I can catch them if I want to. I knew where to go and I stayed there patiently until the buck came near. I can communicate

psychically with animals. I said to it, 'I'm going to kill you' and it turned its head because it knew I had it." [Daly]

After taking Androctonus, this hunter became much calmer and happier. His severe allergies and headaches disappeared, his arthritis was greatly ameliorated, and his blood sugar problems and high blood pressure were lessened considerably ("My doctor said to me, 'What happened?'"). He also became less interested in his extensive collection of knives and guns.

Androctonus is just one of many animal poisons that have become indispensable homeopathic remedies. Other poison remedies include snake venoms — invaluable remedies during menopause and for heart disease — and spider remedies like *Tarentula*, a remedy that is often used for hyperactive children. Of course, all of these remedies are given in highly dilute doses.

Animal remedies have also been derived from other, less obvious sources. For example, remedies made from sea animals include: *Sepia* (ink of the cuttlefish); *Homarus* (lobster); *Ambra Grisea* (a secretion of the sperm whale); and *Spongia Tosta* (roasted sponge). Another important class of animal remedies are those made from mammal milks, including: dog's milk, cat's milk, dolphin's milk, goat's milk, lion's milk, wolf's milk, monkey's milk, and human milk (a powerful remedy that has been successfully used in cases of severe mental illness).

One of the very first milk remedies to be proved was *Lac Caninum* or dog's milk. Its symptoms, especially its mental symptoms, reflect the situation of the domesticated dog. Rajan Sankaran writes:

> "This remedy has in it the nature of the dog, an animal that has been totally controlled and civilized so that it has to suppress its basic nature... It is dependent on its master for food and so it is out to please him. Its survival depends upon keeping its master happy by its performance, its affection, etc. It has to perform or it won't be wanted anymore and its master will kick it out... But the dog knows that no matter how much it tries to please, it will never be equal to the human. It feels inferior, knows that it is at the bottom of the hierarchy... The animal side is also malicious... They can be quite aggressive and defensive... The main

theme of Lac Caninum [the remedy] is dominance... and who is going to be on top. Lac Caninum persons can be irritable and ferocious, but if someone is more irritable and ferocious, they give up, they submit. Then arises the conflict within themselves: 'Do I want to be what I am?' They develop a feeling of low self-worth: 'I am not good enough. I feel dirty and horrible,' and become contemptuous of themselves... They try hard to please, to be liked, cared for and accepted because they feel left out and rejected. They can develop malice and hatred because they hold somebody else responsible for their condition." [Sankaran97, p. 109]

Sankaran points out that the Lac Caninum state can arise in a person as the result of societal racism, child abuse, or being a child in a home where other children are preferred for being better looking. For whatever reason, whether real or imagined, a person in a Lac Caninum state feels that they are inherently deficient and unacceptable. Moreover, they sense that there is nothing they can do about it — their situation is not their own fault, but rather, lies in others' judgment of them. Certainly, the derisive use of the word "bitch" in our society says a lot about our collective subconscious view of the female dog. Isn't it astounding that ingesting an infinitesimal potentized dose of dog's milk could cause a prover to develop these kinds of feelings? And that a dose of dog's milk could cure a person experiencing these same feelings?

On the physical plane, other symptoms of Lac Caninum also echo dog-related themes. Like the dog, Lac Caninum patients feel better out in the open air and from drinking cold drinks. They tend to be nervous, oversensitive, restless, and can suffer from prostration. One of the most important spheres of action for Lac Caninum is the throat, which can be sore, red, and glistening, or covered with white patches. In fact, Lac Caninum had one of its first significant uses as a curative remedy for a diphtheria epidemic. Swallowing and talking can be difficult in Lac Caninum cases, and there may be profuse salivation and drooling. Being derived from milk, it is also not surprising that Lac Caninum (like most milk remedies) has effects upon the female genital organs. Patients may have menstrual periods that are too early, hot, and gushing. They can also have severely swollen and painful breasts before menstruation, and dried up or scanty milk while nursing.

PLANTS AND MINERALS, TOO

It is amazing enough that animal remedies seem to echo themes so obviously related to their source material. But the same is true for plant and mineral remedies. A few years ago, one of my homeopathy teachers began class by showing us a video of lava pouring out of a volcano. He asked us to volunteer our impressions; what did we think the state of lava might be like? How does it "feel" as it erupts, flows, hardens, and meets the sea? Words came to us such as "hot," "relentless," "unstoppable."

Next, the instructor described the results of a blind proving of lava. Even though the provers didn't know what substance they were testing, some of them had sensations of intense heat the moment the remedy hit their tongue! Others developed the feeling of being carried away by some force, as though nothing could stop them. One prover, who was by nature very quiet and demure, became so unfeeling and strident that she just blatantly began to say whatever she wanted at all times. Another prover experienced dreams of falling off an abyss, with bits and pieces of herself being knocked off as she descended — just as one might imagine lava fragmenting and hardening as it falls off a cliff into the sea. This was a powerful lesson to all of us about the mysterious nature of the doctrine of signatures.

SYMBOLISM AND STRUCTURE

The world of homeopathy today is burgeoning with efforts to better understand remedy symptom patterns and themes, and to utilize this information clinically. In recent years, many homeopaths have begun to examine families of remedies, with the hope that related remedies will manifest similar themes. As it turns out, this has been largely borne out.

Homeopathic remedy families are usually based on natural concepts such as groupings of related animals and plants. Thus it is common today to see homeopathy workshops given on the "Sea Remedies," "Conifer Remedies," "Sunflower Remedies," "Snake Remedies," "Milk Remedies," etc. Each of the remedies in these families exhibits similar symptom patterns and themes. For example, most snake remedies tend to be hot, talkative, jealous, and suffer from circulatory problems. Once the themes of a family are understood, they can provide useful clues for remedy selection. For example, if a patient is extremely loquacious, jealous of her spouse, and suffers from high blood pressure and hot flashes, a homeopath will likely determine that she is a candidate for a snake remedy. The patient's case can then be analyzed in more detail in order to select the best matching snake.

This strategic use of families enables today's homeopaths to broaden the range of remedies they can effectively use. Though the homeopaths of the 1800s recognized many kinds of relationships between remedies, they tended to study and understand each remedy one at a time. Unfortunately, most people can master only one or two hundred remedies in this way. If, however, a homeopath can master 100 remedy families, each with about 10 remedies in it, they can expand their effective knowledge to 1,000 remedies. Thus, a snakelike patient of the past would most likely have received *Lachesis* — the most commonly used snake remedy. Today, a homeopath is more likely to say to herself, "This looks like a snake remedy. But which one? Maybe it's *Crotalus Horridus* (rattlesnake) or *Cenchris* (copperhead)?"

Of course, animals and plants are fairly easy to cluster into groups because they belong to natural biological families. But homeopaths have also found ways to cluster remedies made from minerals and other elements. A prominent theoretician in this area is Dutch homeopath Jan Scholten, MD, who has popularized the notion that remedies made from elements in the same row or the same column of the periodic table tend to have symptoms in common [Scholten]. Other types of groupings include the metal remedies, the noble gases, and salt families such as the sodium salts or potassium salts. Each of these families has its own distinctive symptom themes and characteristics.

Clearly, this realm of exploration is as broad and fascinating as nature itself. But for now, let's take a step back in time again, to the 1800s. The next chapter will take you on a short guided tour of the development of homeopathy — how it evolved from Hahnemann's discovery of the Law of Similars to the many methods and ideas that exist in the homeopathic world of today.

CHAPTER 6

✣

THE DEVELOPMENT AND EVOLUTION OF HOMEOPATHIC PRACTICE

"The highest ideal of cure is the rapid, gentle and permanent restoration of health; that is, the lifting and annihilation of the disease in its entire extent in the shortest, most reliable, and least disadvantageous way, according to clearly realizable principles."

— SAMUEL HAHNEMANN, MD, Aphorism 2,
Organon of the Medical Art, 1810 [Hahnemann]

IN CHAPTER 2 YOU LEARNED ABOUT HAHNEMANN, THE FOUNDER of homeopathy, and his discovery of the Law of Similars. But that was only the beginning. While Hahnemann planted the seeds from which homeopathy sprang (and, indeed, much of his work is still being unearthed and incorporated into current practice), the homeopathic medical system continued to develop and expand after Hahnemann's death in 1843.

Over the past two centuries, homeopaths have confronted nearly every imaginable disease in almost every possible context. They have treated infants, children, adults, and the elderly; those with chronic disease and those with acute disease; the mentally ill; birthing women; and animals. In the cholera, typhoid, scarlet fever, and flu epidemics of the 19th and early 20th centuries, homeopaths were usually much more successful than their allopathic counterparts. The same was true of homeopathic treatment of venereal disease and tuberculosis. At the turn of the 20th century, many British and American homeopaths were even having success in treating a variety of cancers.

Today, at the dawn of a new millennium, homeopathy is practiced all over the world. It is most prevalent in Europe, India, and Pakistan. But it is also well-known all over South and Central America, Cuba, Mexico, Australia, New Zealand, Malaysia, Israel, and South Africa. Homeopathy has also developed an increasingly large presence in Eastern Europe and Russia and, of course, is undergoing a rejuvenation in Canada and the United States.

With the passage of time and homeopathy's spread worldwide, homeopathic practitioners have developed a multiplicity of methods. In Europe, homeopathic methodology ranges from the polypharmacy of France, where low-potency combination remedies are used, to the more classical single-remedy homeopathy of the United Kingdom. In the United States, we have naturopaths who combine homeopathy with herbalism, acupuncturists who combine homeopathy with Chinese medicine, and classical homeopaths who practice much like their counterparts in England. This same spectrum can be found in other English-speaking countries like Canada, Australia, and New Zealand. In South America, homeopathic physicians have successfully experimented with massive programs of homeopathic "vaccination" — i.e., the use of remedies as prophylaxis against disease, in lieu of traditional vaccines.

Interestingly, the most intensive and widespread use of homeopathy in the world today is probably taking place in India, where a whole system of homeopathic medical schools exists and licensed practitioners can treat in full hospital settings. Each day, the bustling clinics of India treat hundreds of patients suffering from just about any disease — meningitis, tuberculosis, even leprosy. Several Indian homeopaths have also become known for their experience in treating cancer. This kind of treatment for cancer is nearly impossible in the United States because of laws that limit cancer treatment to surgery, radiation, and chemotherapy. Indian homeopaths have also had astonishing success in treating patients with HIV — so much so, that the Indian government has begun to take notice and invest more research money in their work [India].

HAHNEMANN'S DEVELOPMENT OF THE HOMEOPATHIC SYSTEM

So how did we get here — from Hahnemann to the homeopathic world of today? It all began with Hahnemann's unwavering goal: to attain an ideal form of cure — one that was rapid, gentle, permanent, and reliable. All the work he did to further develop the homeopathic system was motivated by this medical ideal.

Of course, the crude medical practices of Hahnemann's time were anything but gentle and reliable. And when Hahnemann began his practice of homeopathy, his cures, though perhaps more rapid and reliable than those of his allopathic counterparts, also lacked gentleness. Don't forget, he was using mostly poisonous substances, and he had not yet begun to experiment with high dilutions. While undiluted remedies could bring about cure if their application was homeopathic, they could also cause difficult aggravations. Although such reactions were accepted by the patients of that time (who, after all, were accustomed to being bled and taking toxic doses of mercury and opiates), they were not acceptable to Hahnemann. Being a man who believed that God would not have placed humanity on Earth only to suffer, he was confident that a better way existed. He only needed to find it.

For the last 40 years of his life, Hahnemann experimented with every possible method of applying the Law of Similars that he could think of. He tried many new ways of preparing medicines (diluting and potentizing them to various degrees and in various ways); methods of dosing (varying dosage amounts and repetitions of dose); and avenues of administration (dry pills, liquid, inhalation, and external application). He also experimented with a variety of remedy sequences. In so doing, he discovered many kinds of relationships that exist between remedies — for example, that certain remedies tend to follow one another well, while others have negative interactions. Along the way, Hahnemann also continued to develop and test new remedies so that he could build up his underlying repertoire of treatment options. Let's look at some of these developments now in more detail. (If you are not interested in the specifics of homeopathic practice, you can safely skim this chapter or move directly to Chapter 7 or Chapter 8.)

POTENTIZATION — THE CREATION OF THE ULTRADILUTE REMEDIES

Once Hahnemann convinced himself of the utility of the Law of Similars, he began to try and make its application more gentle. The most obvious strategy was to lessen the doses of medicine he gave to his patients. At first, he simply tried to dilute his remedies, usually in a mixture of water and alcohol. But eventually, they had no effect. Being a chemist, he then tried to make sure that these dilutions were truly well-mixed. He did this by *succussing* or vigorously shaking them. Hahnemann found this to have an incredible effect. Not only did the succussed dilutions now work, but they seemed to have even greater curative power than more concentrated doses. In the first edition of the *Organon,* he wrote:

> "There is no small difference in the effects of a dilution which is, as it were, only superficial, and a dilution which is so intimate and uniform that every smallest part of the fluid medium contains a due proportion of the dissolved medicine; the former is much less powerful than the latter." [Hahnemann1stOrganon, Aphorism 250]

Hahnemann came to call this method of preparing medicines, which combines both dilution and succussion, *potentization.* He used this term because he found that this method actually made his remedies more potent. Indeed, it could render otherwise nonmedicinal substances medicinal. For example, foods such as onion, garlic, salt, cinnamon, asparagus, tomato, potato, and milk become powerful remedies when potentized.

Of course, being a chemist, Hahnemann realized that very little if any original substance was likely to be found in these high dilutions. While Avogadro's number — the point at which there is not a single molecule of original substance likely remaining in a dilution — was not established with certainty until 1909, Avogadro's first hypothesis about molecular weight was first made in 1811, about the same time that Hahnemann began to experiment with the higher potencies [Furtsch]. Hahnemann suspected that the effects of potentized remedies were likely not to be biochemical at all — that is, acting on the material body alone. Instead, he hypothesized that they were acting on a more "energetic" or insubstantial plane — what he called the "life principle" or *vital force*, or what the Greeks called the *dynamis*. For this reason, Hahnemann also used the term *dynamization* for potentization. This implied that the dilution and succussion process somehow enabled a remedy substance to reach the dynamic plane.

Hahnemann also experimented with dilution and succussion in a dry medium. He found that a dry medicinal substance could be "diluted" by mixing it with milk-sugar powder and "succussed" by vigorously grinding or *triturating* the two together. In fact, this strategy worked just as well as liquid potentization. Hahnemann surmised that the amazing effects of liquid and dry potentization were due to some kind of friction between the medicinal substance and its diluent, be it liquid or solid:

> "This remarkable alteration in the properties of natural bodies is achieved through mechanical action on their smallest particles by trituration and succussion *while these particles are separated from one another by means of an intervening, indifferent substance that is either dry or liquid*. This procedure develops the latent *dynamic* powers of the substance which were previously unnoticeable, as if slumbering." [Hahnemann, Aphorism 269]

It has taken nearly two hundred years for science to catch up with Hahnemann. Recent physics and medical experiments have been able to demonstrate that succussion is indeed the key to potentization; without this step, a high-potency liquid dilution is merely water. Although potentized ultradilutions may not contain even a single molecule of original substance, they have now been shown to contain some kind of residual energetic signature that can cause the same changes in living tissue that the original substance could cause [Benveniste88, Elia, Ennis].

The ramifications of this discovery are astounding. Just think about it. A very small amount of medicinal substance could yield, via potentization, billions of effective doses! Imagine how the pharmaceutical industry would be impacted if expensive drugs could be used in this way; a very small amount of medicine could yield low-cost doses for everyone on the planet. Given the potential financial consequences, this work is controversial to say the least. Researchers who work on ultradilutions are routinely ridiculed and debunked. But they have persisted and have returned with more confirmatory results.

Interestingly, most of the research on ultradilutions is not being done by homeopaths. In fact, many of the scientists involved in this area know very little about homeopathy as a medical system. Instead, their goal is to create other kinds of potentized substances, such as potentized allopathic drugs. It is fascinating, however, that many of their discoveries have confirmed those made by Hahnemann two hundred years ago. For example, they have found that extreme heat can diminish the effects of a dilution — as did Hahnemann. Chapter 7 will discuss these experimental results in greater detail and will also present several modern clinical trials of homeopathy.

THE CENTESIMAL, DECIMAL, AND LM POTENCIES

In his efforts to create gentle and effective remedies, Hahnemann experimented with a variety of dilution ratios and amounts of succussion. He found that one of the most effective dilution ratios was 1:100 — i.e., 1 unit of medicinal substance combined with 99 units of diluent. This ratio yields the *centesimal* or "c" potencies. Another common dilution ratio, 1:10, yields the *decimal* or "x" potencies (also called "D" potencies). The decimal potencies were first introduced in 1838 by both a German homeopath, Vehsmayer, and an American homeopath named Dubs. However, this dilution ratio did not come into vogue until well after Hahnemann's death.

To give you a better idea of how homeopathic dilutions are created, let's go through the process in more detail. Suppose that we wanted to create a 3c potency of Arnica. We would start with a *mother tincture* of the Arnica flower. Usually, tinctures are made by placing a flower directly into a vial of alcohol; in other cases, the substance is ground up or its juice is squeezed out. Each homeopathic remedy is associated with precise instructions for the creation of its mother tincture. These instructions must be followed by all pharmacies that abide by the homeopathic pharmacopoeia of their country. In the United States, we have Homeopathic Pharmacopoeia of the U.S. (HPUS), which was first published in 1882 and was given formal legal status in 1938, via the same legislation that created the Food and Drug Administration (FDA) [Winston, p. 234].

After creation of an Arnica mother tincture, the potentization process continues by combining 1 drop of tincture with 99 drops of diluent (a mixture of alcohol and water). This mixture is then vigorously shaken by hand, typically by striking it against a surface between 2 and 100 times. Today, machines are sometimes used instead of hand succussion. Once succussion is complete, the 1c potency of Arnica has been created. To create the next higher potency, the process is repeated — but using the preceding potency solution instead of the mother tincture. Thus, combining 1 drop of Arnica 1c solution with 99 drops of diluent, followed by succussion, yields the 2c potency of Arnica. Then, mixing 1 drop of Arnica 2c solution with 99 drops of diluent followed by succussion yields the 3c potency. And so on.

If a remedy is made from insoluble material, it is potentized by *triturating* or grinding it with milk sugar. Thus, instead of mixing 1 drop of remedy or tincture with 99 drops of water and alcohol, 1 unit of solid matter is ground into 99 units of milk sugar. The succussion step is then replaced by one hour of grinding. Hahnemann found that nearly any dry substance — even insoluble substances — could be successfully dissolved in liquid once they had been triturated up to the 3c potency. Thereafter, higher potencies could be created via liquid dilution and succussion.

Now, if you do the math, you will find that potentization quickly yields dilutions in excess of Avogadro's number (approximately 10^{23}). This point has already been passed by the time a 12c or 24x potency has been made — i.e., a dilution of 100^{12} or 10^{24}. Homeopaths call potencies below this threshold *material doses*, because there is still some possibility that some of the original material exists within them. Potencies above this threshold are called *nonmaterial* or *dynamic* doses.

Naturally, the use of nonmaterial doses has always been controversial and sometimes a source of ridicule — even in the time of Hahnemann. The issue has caused infighting among homeopaths themselves over the past two hundred years. In the early 1900s, for example, most of the American allopathic-homeopaths used only material doses. Hahnemann himself was also skeptical of higher potencies in his early years as a homeopath. Initially, he favored potencies such as 3c, 6c, 9c, and 12c. Later on, however, he began to favor 18c, 24c, and 30c, simply because he found them to be more effective. In the last 10 years of his life, he began to experiment with doses as high as 200c. Eventually, potencies as high as 1,000c (also called 1M), 10,000c (10M), 50,000c (50M), and 100,000c (CM) became popular, especially in the United States. These extremely high potencies were popularized by James T. Kent, MD, an American homeopath of the late 1800s, and were produced using specially designed machines. Today, the use of these ultrahigh potencies is common and well-accepted by nearly all homeopaths.

Near the end of his life, Hahnemann devised one more potency scale as a complement to the centesimal potencies. These are the LM potencies, created using a dilution ratio of 1:50,000. (LM potencies are sometimes called "Q" potencies, because of the Latin term *quinquagintamillesimal*, which means "1 in 50,000.") Hahnemann developed LM potencies to be used in conjunction with a liquid dosing regimen, which I will describe in the next section. But because a description of them did not appear in the *Organon* until its last (sixth) edition, which remained unpublished until 1921, they remained unknown to homeopaths of the late 19th and early 20th centuries. As a result, the homeopathic system that spread around the world during that period focused solely on the use of centesimal and decimal potencies. Today, LM potencies are finally coming into greater use.

REMEDY ADMINISTRATION: HOW, HOW MUCH, AND HOW OFTEN

Once he created a potentized remedy dilution, Hahnemann applied small drops of it to tiny sugar pellets and let them dry. These are the little white pills that homeopathy is known for. Up until the time of the fourth edition of the *Organon* in 1829, Hahnemann always administered his remedies in this pill form — the *dry dose*.

Hahnemann's ideal, of course, was to use the least amount of medicine necessary to cure: the *minimum dose*. This meant that the number of pills used for each dose and the frequency of dosing was to be minimized. Indeed, Hahnemann found that frequent dosing was often unnecessary and sometimes ill-advised. If a remedy was repeated too frequently or too soon, beneficial effects could be undone, or a patient could develop unnecessary aggravations.

For this reason, Hahnemann's use of the dry dose followed a kind of "wait and watch" approach. A single dose was given and the patient's symptoms were closely watched. Based on the nature of a patient's response, Hahnemann could determine if the remedy was correct or incorrect, and, if correct, whether the dose was too high or too low in potency. In general, *another dose of the remedy would not be given until the effects of the previous dose had worn off* — i.e., until symptoms began to return. Repeat doses of a remedy might be of the same potency, or the potency might be adjusted upward or downward based on patient response.

Hahnemann's "wait and watch" approach has always been hard for many patients to accept. In the treatment of chronic disease, the effects of a single 200c dose can sometimes last for months; the effects of a 30c dose, for weeks. When patients are accustomed to taking pills every day (or several times a day) for their maladies, taking a single pill and waiting weeks for another dose may seem a bit strange. But if a patient is sensitive to a remedy, frequent repetitions of a high-potency dry dose can lead to aggravations.

This phenomenon (as well as our modern tendency to overdose ourselves with medications) was used to literary effect in a recently published novel [Bohjalian]. The main character is a lawyer who is treated by a classical homeopath and is cured of his chronic cough with the remedy *Arsenicum Album* (arsenic trioxide). Unfortunately, under the misconception that "more is better," the lawyer surreptitiously takes a vial of the remedy from the homeopath's office. After popping pill after pill, he soon develops a full-blown proving of Arsenicum. Of course, according to modern chemistry, this vial did not contain even a single molecule of arsenic. Nevertheless, the lawyer is soon jittery, anxious, restless, suspicious, and feels tingling in his soles and palms — all symptoms of Arsenicum. Once the homeopath discovers what has happened, she urges him to discontinue his pill popping — and all of his symptoms soon disappear. This story certainly underscores the importance of not self-treating for serious conditions, not taking remedies indiscriminately (they aren't vitamins!), and seeking out a trained practitioner who knows what they're doing.

Of course, sometimes frequent repetition of a remedy *is* called for. It all depends. In acute ailments such as ear infections or the flu, the body uses up a remedy faster and may require more frequent repetitions, even of high potencies. Lower potencies, which tend to cause less aggravations in sensitive or weak patients, are also generally used more frequently. In all cases, however, it is important that the treating homeopath be made aware of both negative and positive responses to a remedy so that appropriate adjustments can be made. In contrast to the use of allopathic drugs, there are no fixed dosing regimens in homeopathy; a great deal depends on a patient's individual response. I have even seen a long-lasting and comprehensive cure of chronic disease take place with a single 12c dose.

Unfortunately, even with his "wait and watch" approach, Hahnemann continued to see aggravations in some of his most sensitive patients. Because he wanted to achieve painless and effective cures for all, his experiments continued. Shortly after the publication of the fourth edition of the *Organon* in 1829, Hahnemann began to try a new strategy — administering remedies in liquid form. He simply placed one or more remedy pills in a small amount of water. The patient could then take more frequent doses (usually a teaspoonful) from this solution after succussing or stirring it. Hahnemann found this approach to be highly successful. It embodied a more gradual way of stimulating a sensitive patient's vital force, with smaller, more frequent nudges toward health. Eventually, he also came to believe that liquid dosing was a more natural way for the energy of a remedy to enter the body.

During the remaining 14 years of his life, Hahnemann experimented with every possible parameter of the liquid dosing method: using a differ-ent number of pills to create a remedy solution; adjusting the size of the solution; varying the number of succussions before each dose; and varying the number of teaspoons to be taken. He also found that succussing the solution before each dose raised its potency slightly. This caused the doses being taken by a patient to be gradually increased in potency over time. Hahnemann felt that this gradual increase enabled the fastest and most gentle cures of all.

Hahnemann applied the principle of the minimum dose to liquid dosing as well. This meant that the minimum number of pills should be used to create a solution, the minimum number of succussions should be applied, the minimum number of teaspoons should be given, and the minimum number of repetitions of dose should be used. If a stronger effect was required, these parameters could be increased; decreasing them helped to remove aggravations. Indeed, Hahnemann found that a remedy solution could be diluted even further if it was required. He developed the practice of using *dilution glasses* — the dose taken from the medicinal solution bottle was diluted in yet another glass of water (a dilution glass), and the dosage amount given to the patient was admin-istered from the dilution glass instead. This step could then be repeated again and again, using successive dilution glasses, if it was necessary for an extremely sensitive patient. Thus, in liquid dosing, Hahnemann final-ly found his most adaptable strategy for attaining rapid, gentle, and reli-able cures.

A description of liquid dosing made its first appearance in the fifth edition of the *Organon* in 1833. At this time, Hahnemann was still using centesimal potencies in liquid. But when he moved to Paris with his new wife Melanie, he was reinvigorated once again (at the age of 78) to begin experimenting anew. While the liquid doses worked well in most cases, he found that low centesimal potencies were sometimes too weak and high centesimal potencies were at times too strong. To deal with this, Hahnemann first experimented with a new method of administration — *olfaction* (inhalation). This method required a patient to take a deep sniff of the remedy. Olfaction did turn out to be effective, but the remedial effects of inhaled doses were usually not as long-lasting.

Eventually, Hahnemann decided to devise a new dilution ratio more suited to liquid dosing. The result was the LM (or Q) potencies — created by using a dilution rate of 1:50,000. He wrote:

> "This method of dynamization, I have found after many laborious experiments and counter-experiments, to be the most powerful and at the same time the mildest in action, as the material part of the medicine is lessened with each dynamization 50,000 times and yet incredibly increased in power." [Hahnemann, Footnote 270g]

One of the most powerful aspects of LM dosing is the flexibility and adjustability of the liquid dosing method. Of course, liquid dosing can also be a bit daunting and complex to patients, at least initially. It requires more communication between homeopath and patient as well, so that an optimal dosing regimen can be achieved. Nevertheless, in my experience, liquid dosing is easy once it has been done a few times.

Another important and distinctive aspect of LM dosing is how LM potencies are used in sequence over time. While centesimal potencies are typically sequenced in large jumps (for example, a patient may first be given a 12c, then a 30c, and later a 200c), LM doses are usually given in a gradually increasing arc of potencies — LM1, LM2, LM3, etc. Since the remedy solution is also succussed a bit before each administration (thereby slightly raising its potency), this strategy truly achieves Hahnemann's ideal of a gradual increase in potency each time the remedy is given. In fact, it was this dosing regimen that we followed daily with Max. Over the course of his first year on the remedy, we progressed up the potency scale from LM1 to LM13, changing from one potency to the next about once a month.

POTENCY SELECTION

The criterion for selecting a patient's remedy is fairly well-defined in homeopathy — pick the remedy whose symptoms best match those of the patient. But how is potency selected? And how often should a dose be repeated? Answers to these questions are much less well-defined. Indeed, I have found that every homeopathic practitioner seems to have their own personal ideas about dosing. Some use the dry-dose "wait and watch" approach exclusively. Others repeat dry doses frequently and routinely, even in high potencies. Many homeopaths are beginning to use LM dosing as well. However, there are a few guidelines that are generally accepted by most homeopaths:

- The more certain you are that you have selected the correct remedy, the higher the potency.

- For mental/emotional symptoms, favor higher potencies; for chronic physical symptoms, favor lower potencies.

- For young, vigorous people, use higher potencies; for older, weaker people, use lower potencies.

- For acute diseases with strong symptoms, use higher potencies.

- For people who are very sensitive (for example, those who suffer from severe allergies), use lower potencies or LM potencies.

- If a patient is on allopathic drugs or there is some part of their routine that is likely to interfere with the action of a remedy, use LM potencies, liquid dosing, or repeated dry doses of low potencies.

One way of unifying all of these rules together is with the following principle: *match the potency of the remedy to the vitality of the patient*. In other words, the higher the vitality of the patient, the higher the potency. The lower the vitality, the lower the potency. This principle unifies the others because each of the other principles can be explained in terms of it.

For example, if a person has a very high vitality, they are likely to develop more well-defined, clear symptoms. As a result, their remedy picture will be clearer and they will get a higher potency. People with a higher vitality also tend to develop mental and emotional symptoms along with their physical symptoms, and sometimes even before physical symptoms appear; they get a higher potency too. In contrast, people with severe physical pathology and few mental or emotional symptoms have often taken a great deal of allopathic drugs; they get lower potencies. Finally, if a person is extremely sensitive to their environment or is routinely taking allopathic drugs that potentially weaken their system or lessen the effects of a homeopathic remedy, they are also likely to have a lowered vitality; they get lower potencies too.

ONE REMEDY AT A TIME

As I have already mentioned, Hahnemann experimented not only with potency and dosing, but with remedy sequences as well. At one point, he even tried using small combinations of remedies. In the end, however, Hahnemann held firmly that remedy combinations should never be used. Even if it was sometimes necessary to alternate or change remedies quickly (even on the same day), he felt that two different remedies should never be used at the same time. In the last edition of the *Organon* he wrote:

> "In no case of cure is it necessary to employ more than a single simple medicinal substance at one time with a patient. For this reason alone, it is inadmissible to do so. It is inconceivable that there could be the slightest doubt about whether it is more in accordance with nature and more reasonable to prescribe only a single, simple well-known medicinal substance at one time in a disease or a mixture of several different ones. In homeopathy — the only true and simple, the only natural medical art — it is absolutely prohibited to administer to the patient, at one time, two different medicinal substances." [Hahnemann, Aphorism 273]

Why such vehemence? Just as it is today, it was common practice in Hahnemann's time for allopathic physicians to prescribe drug mixtures. Often, the contents of these medicines were known only to the pharmacies. Hahnemann felt that these medicinal concoctions were quite dangerous. He spoke out publicly against them and also about the lack of hygiene evident in their manufacture. But because drug mixtures were so popular, it was quite tempting for homeopaths of Hahnemann's time to mix homeopathic remedies together, especially if several different remedies seemed to be likely candidates for a patient. Hahnemann's experiments, however, demonstrated that this practice was simply unnecessary.

As was characteristic for him, Hahnemann's rationale for using only one remedy at a time was fundamentally scientific. First of all, he felt that it was simply impossible to know what the effects of a combination remedy would be without actually proving it as a distinct substance. The Law of Similars states what effects a single proven remedy will have. It says nothing about a combination of remedies. If Hahnemann really wanted to try out a combination substance as a possible remedy, he proved it as a distinct entity. One such remedy was *Hepar Sulphuris Calcareum*, made from a mixture of sulphur and calcium. However, the sulphur and calcium were first combined under extreme heat and pressure to form a distinct material substance. This substance was then potentized and proved as a single remedy so that its precise effects could become known.

Even more important to Hahnemann, however, was the fact that it was impossible to accurately assess the response of a patient to a combination medicine. Which constituent remedy was having the curative effect? What effects were each of the constituent remedies having and how did they interact? Did they interfere with one another? How should treatment proceed if a combination failed? Hahnemann felt that it was important to try one remedy at a time and see if it worked. If it did not, he could then try another remedy, based on the new symptom picture.

Despite Hahnemann's edicts, the principle of the single remedy became a contentious one in homeopathy, and it remains so to this day.

During Hahnemann's lifetime, there were already many homeopaths who used combination remedies. Combinations were also popular in 19th-century America. One of the first American pharmacists to sell them was Frederick Humphreys, MD, a graduate of the Homeopathic Medical College of Pennsylvania. In 1855, his membership in both the American Institute of Homeopathy and the New York State Homeopathic Medical Society was withdrawn because of his manufacture and sale of these combinations. However, his remedies continued to be popular and lucrative. Indeed, as Julian Winston reports in his history of American homeopathy, "Humphreys veterinary products were used by the Ringling Brothers Circus throughout the 1930s and, according to the United States Department of Interior, by the United States Calvary." [Winston, p. 85]

Today, combinations are the mainstay of many French homeopaths, who utilize standardized combinations for specific diseases and as well as combinations that are formulated on an individualized basis. Combinations are also immensely popular in the burgeoning natural health product industry. Even mainstream pharmaceutical companies have begun to market over-the-counter remedy combinations for common ailments such as hay fever, insomnia, premenstrual tension, arthritis, teething, etc. For the most part, these popular combinations contain only a few low-potency remedies. However, more broad-spectrum combinations are starting to be sold that include remedies in very high potencies. For example, one combination recommended for "skin problems" that is now sold by a major pharmacy contains 23 different remedies, some in very high potencies. Other combination formulas I have seen include remedies that are known to be harmful when used together, or are actually known to antidote or nullify one another. It is unfortunate that these concoctions are marketed under the banner of "homeopathy." Naturally, they are also quite alarming to most homeopaths.

So why use mixed remedies (*polypharmacy*) at all? In general, there are two different kinds of thinking behind this practice. In *individualized polypharmacy*, a set of remedies is chosen based on a patient's symptoms. If the practitioner cannot find a single remedy that matches a patient, a few remedies are given in combination, each of which covers different aspects of their case. These combinations usually contain only a small set of remedies (two or three) and are based on the past therapeutic experience of the homeopath, who is (hopefully) also aware of possible remedy interactions.

The other approach to polypharmacy, exemplified by over-the-counter combinations, is non-individualized *disease-based polypharmacy*. In this case, a set of remedies is chosen, all of which are known to have some relationship to the targeted condition or disease — for example, hay fever. These remedies are thrown together with the idea that one of them will cure — a "shotgun" approach.

Since disease-based combinations are sold or prescribed without attention to the specific symptoms of an individual patient, they are usually only loosely homeopathic to a patient's disease. As a result, while such products can be helpful, they are usually merely palliative or suppressive — much like allopathic medicines. One proof of this is that combination remedies must often be taken on an ongoing basis and that symptoms return after they are discontinued. This is not surprising; since disease-based combinations are only superficially homeopathic to a patient, their effect is only superficial as well. The danger in their use is the same as the danger inherent in the use of over-the-counter allopathic medicines. If a person takes them for an extended period of time, they may permanently suppress their symptoms, leading to the same kinds of chronic disease that allopathic medicines can cause.

Despite the fact that classical homeopaths consider combination remedies to be a substandard form of treatment, such remedies are, nevertheless, quite popular. On the bright side, these products help to popularize homeopathy and eventually convince many people to seek out more suitable professional homeopathic treatment. Indeed, if a combination remedy contains only a few well-selected low-potency remedies and is only used for a short period of time, it is usually beneficial and benign. But treatment under the care of a qualified homeopath is always preferable and will generally be more effective.

RELATED APPLICATIONS AND METHODS

If you are currently under the care of a homeopath, you may have discovered that they use techniques that I have not yet mentioned. Some of them may be quite classical and "Hahnemannian"; others less so. Indeed, even the most classical practitioner uses alternative strategies from time to time. For the remainder of this chapter, I will describe some of the more commonly used methods that lie outside of the basic homeopathic paradigm. I include this information because I believe it is important for everyone to understand the rationale behind the treatments they use. It is also important for patients to understand which treatment methods are actually "homeopathy" and which are not.

Homeopathic Prophylaxis for Acute Disease

I have already discussed the traditional homeopathic approach to treating and preventing epidemic disease. This approach was outlined by Hahnemann himself. As early as 1801, he published one of his first essays on the homeopathic method entitled "Cure and Prevention of Scarlet Fever." He discovered that in a particular epidemic of scarlet fever, the remedy *Belladonna* (made from the deadly nightshade plant) was effective in not only curing the fever, but it could also be used as a prophylactic to prevent the disease entirely.

As described in Chapter 4, to determine the appropriate remedies for treating and preventing an epidemic disease, homeopaths combine the symptoms of several afflicted people together to create "the case of the epidemic." The small set of remedies that match these symptoms is called the *genus epidemicus.* These remedies can then be used to cure those who have been infected, as well as prophylactically — to prevent the disease entirely.

This kind of *homeoprophylaxis* lies well within the Hahnemannian paradigm. A key aspect of the approach is that prophylactic remedies are given only when the threat of disease is imminent and its characteristics are known with certainty. This is very different from today's blanket use of vaccinations, which are given according to a prescribed timetable, even when the threat of disease is negligible. Allopathic vaccination also uses the disease virus itself as the prophylactic agent. This is not usually true of homeopathic prophylaxis; the genus epidemicus rarely includes the remedy made from the disease matter itself.

Another important difference between homeoprophylaxis and vaccination is that the remedies suitable for one particular instance of an epidemic (for example, a whooping cough epidemic) may be different from the remedies suitable for another instance of the same type of epidemic. This is true because each epidemic has its own unique characteristics and symptoms. Because the remedies that will be useful for a future epidemic cannot be precisely determined in advance, most classical homeopaths feel that the best general-purpose prophylactic against infectious disease is ongoing homeopathic treatment. This helps to ensure that a patient is healthy and not susceptible to an epidemic in the first place.

Of course, many homeopathic patients are afraid to forego vaccinations entirely and are eager to find some kind of replacement for them within the homeopathic paradigm. In response, some homeopaths have experimented with the remedies made from disease matter — *nosodes* — as homeopathic "vaccinations." While this practice is not strictly within the confines of classical homeopathy (nosodes do not always cause the symptoms of their respective diseases in provings; in fact, nosodes are usually used to treat other conditions), this method has proven to be effective in many cases. For example, in the early 1900s, when several outbreaks of smallpox were occurring in the United States, *Variolinum* (made from a smallpox pustule) was used successfully to not only prevent smallpox, but to treat it as well. In the state of Iowa, Variolinum was even allowed to be used in lieu of traditional vaccination [Eaton].

Other nosodes that have been used as prophylactics include *Diphtherinum* to prevent diphtheria, *Pertussinum* to prevent pertussis (whooping cough), *Morbillinum* to prevent measles, *Influenzinum* to prevent the flu, and *Anthracinum* to prevent anthrax. Indeed, a homeopathic nosode can be made from disease matter for any disease. Remember, of course, that not even a single molecule of actual disease matter exists within any of these highly potentized remedies. Also note that the use of nosodes to treat (rather than to prevent) a disease should be done with caution. The homeopathic literature of the 1800s, for example, explicitly advised against the use of the nosode *Tuberculinum* in active cases of tuberculosis.

As it turns out, the use of nosodes as prophylactics has been studied experimentally in modern times. One active researcher in this area was the late Francisco Eizayaga, MD, an Argentinian homeopath. Due to his influence, South America has been the scene of several large-scale experiments. For example, in August 1974, there was an epidemic of meningitis in Guaratingueta, Brazil. As part of a trial, 18,640 children were given *Meningococcinum* 10c, while 6,340 children did not receive the nosode. Out of the 18,640 children, only 4 cases of meningitis developed; out of the 6,340 children, 34 cases were noted. The net effect: untreated children had 25 times the chance of contracting the disease than homeopathically treated children [CastroNogueria]. Homeopathic prophylaxis is also popular in Europe for domestic animals — for example, to control bovine mastitis [Spranger] and kennel cough. Two recent studies on homeopathic prophylaxis in animals will be discussed in Chapter 7.

Now that we are in an era in which biological warfare is truly a potential threat, it seems only good common sense that homeopathic methods be given a closer look by the medical establishment. In recent testimony given to Congress on this subject, prominent researchers have specifically recommended homeopathic methods of prophylaxis, not only because they are safer than allopathic vaccines, but because they can be adapted rapidly to unknown diseases as well as to diseases for which no vaccination is available [Jonas01]. For all of these reasons, prejudice must be overcome and financial interests must be ignored; the safety and well-being of the public is at stake.

Isopathy / Tautopathy

The use of disease nosodes to treat or prevent diseases is actually an example of a treatment method closely related to homeopathy called *isopathy.* Isopathy treats disease by using a remedy made from a by-product of the disease or from a substance that seems to have triggered the disease. Another example of this method is the use of potentized allergens to help allergy sufferers. Isopathy is not homeopathy in the strict sense because isopathic remedies have usually not been shown to elicit the targeted symptoms in healthy provers. However, like many therapies that utilize potentized substances, isopathy is closely associated with homeopathy. Indeed, many homeopaths use this approach when other attempts to find the simillimum have failed.

Another practice that is similar to isopathy, but is more in line with classical homeopathic practice, is *tautopathy.* This method utilizes a potentized drug or toxin in order to cure a person who is known to have been poisoned by it. For example, a person who has been poisoned by ongoing use of steroids might be given a homeopathic dose of steroid to help rid the body of its toxic effects. Or, a potentized vaccine might be used to counteract vaccine damage. One amazing example of tautopathy was described by one of my teachers, British homeopath Simon Taffler. He gave potentized *Mercury* to a dental nurse who was showing signs of mercury poisoning. Shortly thereafter, a large amount of mercury was discharged in her menstrual blood. Her body had responded to the homeopathic stimulus by cleansing itself.

Tautopathy is in line with classical homeopathic practice because the patient is indeed experiencing symptoms that are known to be caused by the remedy substance; i.e., tautopathy is clearly an application of the Law of Similars. However, like isopathy, tautopathy is usually used by homeopaths only when other remedies fail to cure. In such cases, the poisoning drug has created a complicating factor that must be eliminated in order for a full cure to take place. Here is a typical example of such a situation, described by British homeopath Ian Watson:

> "A woman in her sixties came to see me and told me her 'gullet had shrunk.' When she tried to swallow, food became lodged behind the sternum, causing a 'hot' pain which went through to the back. The pain was relieved by regurgitating the food. On drinking she often had

spasmodic attacks of hiccoughs. She had frequent eructations [belching] of wind; a sensation of a lump in the throat, not relieved by swallowing; easy satiety and a tendency towards constipation.

About eight years previously she had an internal investigation of the gullet which caused lacerations and punctured her right lung. The lung collapsed and she developed pleurisy as a result. This had left her with a tendency to get out of breath easily, and soreness in the chest on deep inspiration. While I was studying the case I gave *Arnica* 200 [200c] followed by *Calendula* 30 on the basis of the past trauma, and this relieved the soreness in the chest but produced no other change. On repertorising the symptoms *Natrum Muriaticum* [potentized salt] seemed best indicated but it was given with no result. *Kali carbonicum* [potassium carbonate] and *Lachesis* [a snake poison remedy] were also tried but without relief.

I decided to question her for further information about the onset of the trouble. It transpired that approximately one year after the lung episode she had 'an attack of arthritis' in the right hip. She was given Naprosyn (a non-steroid anti-inflammatory drug). As soon as she started taking it she developed the awful burning in the oesophagus. After a week the drug was stopped, but ever since then she had had the difficulty swallowing, pain behind the sternum and feeling of a lump in the throat. In fact, she assured me she had 'never been well since.'

On hearing this I obtained a bottle of *Naprosyn* 30 [the drug Naprosyn potentized up to 30c] and sent her three doses to take over a 24-hour period. The next day her husband called to ask 'What the hell have you given to my wife?' He said she had never looked so ill since the Asian flu thirty years ago! I tried to sound confident that all would be well, and said to wait another day. The next day the woman rang me and proudly declared she had just eaten toast without any problem for the first time in years. She had no further trouble at all for about three months — she could swallow anything, there was no pain or regurgitation, her wind disappeared and her general health improved considerably. Then she had a partial relapse after the sudden death of a close friend, which *Ignatia* 200 [a grief-related remedy] took care of very quickly. I sent further Naprosyn 30... but she never needed to take it." [Watson, pp. 109–110]

Organ Remedies

Another method associated with homeopathy is the use of remedies to strengthen or "cleanse" specific organs. The use of these so-called *organ remedies* is loosely homeopathic because provings have demonstrated their affinity to particular organs. For example, *Chelidonium Majus* (a plant remedy made from celandine, a yellow-flowered herb of the poppy family) is sometimes used for cleansing or strengthening the liver, because its proving symptoms include many symptoms of liver disease — for instance, jaundice and pain under the right shoulder blade. Another kind of organ therapy is called *organotherapy*. This approach uses *sarcodes* — remedies made from healthy organ tissue. For instance, *Thyroidinum*, made from dried sheep's thyroid gland, is sometimes used in cases of thyroid disease.

Homeopaths who routinely use organ remedies believe that they help to reduce aggravations. They are also used in cases in which an organ has been severely damaged or removed. Here is another illustrative case by Ian Watson:

> "I treated a boy who had a brain tumor removed and who recovered generally but his growth was stunted. This was thought due to the tumor having impinged upon his pituitary gland. Constitutional treatment helped him generally but didn't affect his growth, which was the main problem. Consequently, I gave him *Pituitrin* 30... and he started to grow normally soon after starting the remedy." [Watson, p. 59]

In contrast to standard homeopathic treatment, organ remedies are usually prescribed in low doses and are repeated frequently. Often, a mother tincture will be used. For this reason, the use of organ remedies is viewed by many homeopaths as more akin to herbalism than homeopathy. Nevertheless, if the use of these remedies is based on the similarity of a patient's symptoms to proving data, the method does lie within the homeopathic paradigm.

Cell Salts

Very similar in flavor to organotherapy is the use of *cell salt* remedies. These potentized remedies were popularized in 1873 by a German homeopath, Dr. William Schuessler. They are made from mineral salts commonly found in the human body. For example, the remedy *Calcarea Sulphurica*, made from calcium sulphate, is known for its effects on connective tissue. Like organ remedies, cell salts are usually given in low potencies and are repeated frequently. Some homeopaths believe that they help to boost the body's functioning. If they are used because of the similarity of proving symptoms to those being experienced by a patient, their use is homeopathic. If they are used as a kind of health tonic or vitamin, such treatment lies outside the boundaries of classical homeopathy.

Specifics

Some remedies are used with such regularity and with such success for certain conditions that they are called *specifics* for those conditions. Probably the most well-known specific is *Arnica* for trauma-related injuries, which I described in detail in Chapter 5. Not surprisingly, specifics are most often associated with acute conditions. In quick-paced acute diseases (such as trauma and many types of infections), most people develop the same symptoms. If those symptoms match the symptoms of a particular remedy, that remedy will naturally become known as a "specific" for that disease or situation. Other examples of specifics are *Kali Bichromicum* (potassium bichromate) for sinus infections and *Cocculus* (Indian cockle, a plant) or *Tabacum* (tobacco) for motion sickness.

Of course, homeopathic practice is rarely quite as simple as the use of specifics seems to imply. Though people may resort to specifics in a crunch, they are usually not the answer in the long term. For one thing, they do not usually address the underlying problem that is causing a person to experience their symptoms. Why does a person have a tendency to get sinus infections or motion sickness? That is the real problem to be solved.

LOOSELY RELATED METHODS AND MODALITIES

This final section discusses practices that tend to be associated with homeopathy because they use some form of potentized medicine or because they utilize substances that homeopathic remedies are also made from. However, they are not based on the Law of Similars. As a result, they have no real relationship to homeopathy.

Intuitive or "Energy-Reading" Machine Prescribing

Sometimes people approach me with stories that go something like this: "Amy, I went to a 'homeopath.' He used a pendulum to decide on five remedies — a unique combination just for me!" Or, "My chiropractor hooked me up to a machine that tested my energy field and came up with this remedy."

It should be clear to you by now that a remedy chosen on the basis of anything else but a patient's symptoms cannot be considered homeopathy. To my knowledge, no device has ever been proven to measure a patient's energy field and to reliably match it to a remedy.

Of course, some homeopaths do use "intuitive" techniques such as dowsing or applied kinesiology to select a remedy from a set of potential remedy choices. This can be considered in the realm of homeopathy if the initial remedy choices are actually based on the Law of Similars. But if remedy selection is based solely on psychic techniques or "energy-reading machines," it cannot be called homeopathy, even if potentized remedies are ultimately prescribed.

As far as the success of such methods, I have heard that they are palliative at best, rarely truly curative. Some have speculated that good results occur only when a practitioner successfully taps into their own intuition about the correct remedy. Such results are necessarily limited or enhanced by the practitioner's knowledge of materia medica and their understanding of a patient's symptoms. Here's an anecdote from Marybeth Buchele-Moseman, CCH, RSHom (NA). When she wrote this, she was still a student of homeopathy. Today she is a professional homeopath practicing in St. Louis Park, Minnesota and Menomonie, Wisconsin. The quote below describes her initial experience with a "machine" prescriber who treated her for chronic fatigue:

> "The first homeopath I saw did this exact type of treatment, so I'm very familiar with it. That clinic I went to was (is) staffed with MDs

and had a waiting list. They did get results, but the question I would put to you is the question that I did not get a good answer for until I saw a classical homeopath: is this treatment healing the problem or is it just Band-Aiding the symptoms? I used this treatment for over three years, making many... expensive trips out-of-state... because the treatments just patched me up, they never took care of the underlying imbalances that were really making me sick.

I was a very vocal defender of that type of treatment (because I got some results at a time when nothing else was available). But then I experienced classical homeopathy, meaning taking one remedy at a time, the remedy chosen after an extensive interview with the homeopath. With classical homeopathy I have experienced health in the form of freedom and flexibility beyond anything I could have imagined. I am comfortable in my own skin, I look very different and feel very different on the physical level and on the mental-emotional level... The gift and challenge of homeopathy is that even very bad homeopathy gets results of some type. And if a person has been quite sick, with little or no help from the conventional docs, even some results seem better than none. This type of treatment is often (but not always) used by practitioners who are poorly trained, who are looking for shortcuts, who want the income from being able to see a lot of patients in a short time (otherwise known as running a patient-mill clinic)." [MB]

Bach Flower Remedies

Edward Bach, MD, was a British physician of the early 1900s who was introduced to homeopathy around 1919, when he worked as a bacteriologist and pathologist at the London Homoeopathic Hospital. About 10 years later, he became deeply interested in flowers, and by 1930, he left his London practice to wander the countryside looking for flowers that could be used for healing. His selection of flowers was highly intuitive. Bach believed that he could sense the special healing power of each plant.

The use of Bach flower remedies is a useful healing system in its own right and many homeopaths utilize them as an adjunct to their practice of homeopathy. However, Bach flower remedies have not been proved in homeopathic provings, nor is their selection or reputed action based on the Law of Similars. Although they are said to be "potentized" (a term Bach borrowed from homeopathy), the preparation of Bach flower remedies is nothing like that of homeopathic potentization. For all of these reasons, the use of Bach flower remedies is not homeopathy.

Anthroposophic Remedies

Anthroposophic medicine is a healing system developed by Rudolph Steiner (1861–1925) as part of a philosophical system called anthroposophy. You may be familiar with the Waldorf Schools, whose philosophy is also based on Steiner's ideas. Steiner must have been familiar with homeopathy since he based the preparation of his remedies on the homeopathic potentization process. However, like Bach flower remedies, the use of anthroposophic remedies is based on Steiner's intuition, not on the Law of Similars. There is therefore no relationship between anthroposophic medicine and homeopathy.

Herbalism

Many people who are unfamiliar with homeopathy tend to confuse it with *herbalism* — i.e., the use of plant tinctures to treat disease. This confusion is natural, since homeopaths also use plants as the source of many of their remedies. However, unlike herbalists, homeopaths rarely use plants in tincture form; homeopathic remedies are nearly always potentized ultradilutions. Nevertheless, the primary distinction between homeopathy and herbalism is actually the rationale for using a particular remedy or plant tincture. Homeopathy's application of remedies is based on the Law of Similars — i.e., the symptoms caused in provings and their similarity to the symptoms of a patient. In contrast, herbalists choose their remedies based on accumulated folklore and experience. In some cases, of course, the net effect is the same. Through trial and error, people have discovered the healing powers of plants, and in many cases, the plant is actually homeopathic to the targeted ailment.

In most cases, however, the traditional herbal uses of plants are quite different from their use in homeopathy. A good example is St. John's

Wort — a plant that is also the source of the homeopathic remedy *Hypericum*. The tincture of this plant has become an extremely popular herbal remedy for depression. In homeopathy, Hypericum is an important remedy for nerve damage and nerve pain. Of course, on some level, both uses of this plant address problems with the nervous system. But Hypericum would not even be on a homeopath's top-50 list for the treatment of depression.

One might wonder, of course, if herbal products have different effects from homeopathic remedies since they are given in tincture rather than potentized form. This may be the case. Nevertheless, from a homeopathic point of view, the ongoing use of herbal products such as St. John's Wort may simply be palliative and, in some cases, may result in an eventual proving of the substance. Thus, it would not be surprising to a homeopath to find that a person taking St. John's Wort for depression also develops symptoms of Hypericum. These include: a feeling as if one were lifted high in the air and anxiety about falling from heights; a throbbing headache and a feeling of heavy coldness at the top of the head; thirst and nausea, with a feeling of a lump in the stomach; bleeding hemorrhoids; darting pains in the shoulders, pressure along the side of the arm, cramps in the calves, pain in the toes and fingertips, a feeling of crawling in the hands and feet, and general neuritis; asthma worse in foggy weather; and sweating of the scalp with loss of hair. Unfortunately, it is unlikely that someone taking St. John's Wort daily for depression would associate these symptoms with their use of the plant tincture. While herbalism is a valid and important mode of medicine, it should be used with caution and under the guidance of a trained herbalist.

Energy Healing

Homeopathy is just one among several forms of *energy medicine* — systems that focus on the vital force or energy body. Other energy-based therapies include acupuncture and hands-on healing techniques such as Reiki or Quantum Touch [Brennan, Gordon, Stein]. Hahnemann himself was fascinated by hands-on healing; he even discusses such techniques in the

Organon. He also described the benefits of magnet therapy (magnets were also proved as remedies), electrical therapies, hydrotherapy, and massage. However, none of these practices is homeopathy.

Of course, according to conventional scientific thought, it is highly implausible that the vital force exists or that energy healing or ultradilutions could have any effect whatsoever. The next chapter addresses this skepticism head-on — by providing convincing scientific evidence that homeopathy is indeed a genuinely effective medical system.

CHAPTER 7

⁊

SCIENCE AND SKEPTICISM: DOES HOMEOPATHY REALLY WORK?

"Clearly it is irrational to reject a therapy simply because it seems to lack an underlying mechanism of action. Many of the therapies within conventional medicine... are used both safely and expertly despite our lack of understanding concerning how they work. The scientific community must therefore be honest... with itself... Although painful in the short term, this position is scientifically productive and provides an essential countercurrent to the academic and cultural arrogance that appears to pervade some areas of conventional science."

— GEORGE LEWITH, DM, *Alternative Therapies in Health and Medicine,* 1999 [Lewith]

SCIENCE IS THE GOSPEL OF THE MODERN WORLD. EVERY ADVANCE in medicine, if it is to be accepted, must be backed up by a scientific study. And any new technique that is backed up by such a study is readily accepted — if it fits within the medical framework accepted by most scientists.

But the truth is, science has only scratched the surface of the apparent physical reality that surrounds us — let alone subtler realities that may lie beneath its surface. Despite our modern tendency toward scientific arrogance, we actually have a pretty weak grasp on many aspects of our world. This is especially true of the human body. The brain and the immune system, for instance, are still largely mysteries.

Nevertheless, our ignorance hasn't stopped us from developing effective healing techniques. Through trial and error, observation and inference, humanity has developed many therapies that work, even if we don't understand exactly how they do. This is just as true of allopathy as it is of alternative medicine. In fact, it is estimated that only 10 percent to 20 percent of allopathic techniques are proven or supported by solid scientific evidence [OTA]. To say that a system of medicine like homeopathy doesn't work or can't work, simply because it falls outside the scope of our current level of scientific understanding, is hypocritical — and bad science. It is reminiscent of the "experts" of the early 17th century who refused to look through Galileo's telescope to see the four moons of Jupiter because they "knew" that those moons couldn't possibly exist.

Of course, there has always been skepticism about frontier areas of scientific inquiry — areas outside the boundaries of accepted scientific doctrine. Allopathic skepticism about homeopathy is even understandable; after all, homeopathy contradicts many of the basic tenets of allopathy and is threatening to the livelihood of its practitioners. With their predominantly mechanistic and biochemical orientation toward the human body, most allopaths are quite a long way off from accepting the reality of a subtler energy body.

In recent years, however, the tide seems to have turned just a bit. Perhaps the overthrow of the Newtonian view of the universe by Einstein and the new realities of quantum physics have finally enabled some to open their minds. The public's embrace of alternative therapies has also forced the allopathic frontier to expand a bit — even if the motivations have been largely financial. So perhaps it is nearly time for homeopathy to break through. For despite the fact that it is rooted in the 1800s, homeopathy is actually a medicine of the 21st century. Recent scientific studies seem to indicate that the action of homeopathic remedies may really be all about energy and information — realms of inquiry that only now are beginning to take root and grow in the new millennium.

So where to begin? How can scientists approach a phenomenon like homeopathy? The first step is to determine whether the phenomenon truly exists — whether ultradilutions really do have effects. Once a sufficient existence proof is attained, the next step is to try to determine how it works. Of course, even if we don't have the tools to discover the underlying mechanism of a phenomenon, we can still try to understand it better. How can we make it work for us? How does it impact us? Even if we can't discover how gravity, the genetic code, or homeopathic ultradilutions really work, we can still learn a lot about them.

Scientific exploration of the homeopathic phenomenon has been growing steadily over the past two decades. Despite the marginalized status of homeopathy as a medical discipline in the West, extremely meager funding for homeopathic research, and the disdain that inevitably falls upon anyone who decides to explore this realm, science is finally starting to catch up with the discoveries of Hahnemann. This chapter will describe some of these developments in detail. It begins with several recent clinical trials and studies that prove the reality of the homeopathic phenomenon and its utility in treating disease. Next, work in biophysics and physical chemistry is examined that provides glimmers of illumination about homeopathy's underlying mechanism of action. The chapter concludes with a presentation of several models of remedy action that homeopaths have developed over the past two hundred years of homeopathic practice.

EXISTENCE PROOF

If you ask your allopathic doctor whether homeopathy is a valid form of medicine, they are likely to say that "it hasn't been proven scientifically" or that "any effects are due to the placebo effect." However, these statements have already been shown by scientific studies to be false. There have been scores of successful scientific studies of homeopathy in recent years. These studies have collectively demonstrated that not only is the phenomenon of homeopathy real, but it is not due to the placebo effect. In fact, ironically, it was homeopaths who first introduced the idea of a placebo-controlled study. They developed this method back in the mid 1800s in order to fend off naysayers and skeptics [Dean].

Of course, it is not surprising that most doctors are unreceptive to or unaware of growing scientific evidence of homeopathy's efficacy. Not only does homeopathic philosophy represent a revolutionary (and therefore threatening) shift in medical thinking, but the latest homeopathic research is simply less accessible to American allopaths since the vast majority of it is being conducted in Europe and India.

Homeopathic research is also far less abundant than allopathic research. It is largely unfunded or, at best, conducted on a shoestring budget. And even when successful trials are conducted, there is a documented bias against their publication in mainstream medical journals. Indeed, a recent study was conducted specifically to test for this bias. Two papers, identical in form and content, but one reporting the effects of an allopathic drug and the other reporting the effects of the remedy *Sulphur* (potentized sulphur) on a particular condition, were distributed to 400 unsuspecting reviewers. The "allopathic" paper was recommended for publication and was rated as an important work. The "homeopathic" paper was deemed unimportant and was generally not recommended for publication. When the reviewers were asked to rate specific aspects of the study, like method and reliability, they were less biased. Nevertheless, the significance of the homeopathic paper was questioned. The authors of this bias-study concluded that the "lack of open mindedness in the peer review process could affect the introduction of unconventional concepts into medicine." [Hendersen]

The net effect of underfunding and bias is that fewer studies about homeopathy are conducted and published where doctors can learn about them. These factors also lessen the likelihood that existing studies will be replicated — another requirement for scientific support of a new theory. Nevertheless, there are hundreds of studies out there — at least 17 European research studies on Arnica alone. And increasingly, trials of homeopathic remedies are being conducted by established medical scientists who rigorously adhere to accepted methodology — double-blinding, randomization, and placebo-controls. Gradually, a number of study replications are beginning to appear as well.

One of today's active homeopathic researchers is Wayne Jonas, MD, the former director of the Office of Alternative Medicine at the National Institutes of Health (NIH), who left his post at the NIH to study the effects of ultradilutions. He is now director of the Samueli Institute for Information Biology, whose purpose is to explore the inter-action between biological systems and nonmolecular signals — i.e., the kinds of signals that may be transmitted by homeopathic remedies. Jonas is coauthor of a book with Jennifer Jacobs, MD, which describes many recent homeopathic clinical trials [Jonas&Jacobs]. He was also part of a team that conducted a meta-analysis of homeopathic trials that will be described later on in this chapter [Linde].

In 1999, Dr. Jonas published a paper that reported his use of a home-opathic nosode (a remedy made from diseased tissue or a disease by-product) as a prophylactic against infection [Jonas]. This study was conducted on mice in extremely well-controlled laboratory conditions in the Department of Cellular Immunology at Walter Reed Army Institute of Research, located in Rockville, Maryland. The goal of the trial was to test the effects of a nosode prepared from francisella tularen-sis–infected tissue on the mortality of mice later infected with this same deadly organism. Fifteen trials were conducted, each on 142 age-matched male mice. Various different potencies of the nosode were used: 3x, 7x, 14x, 30c, 200c, 1,000c, as well as combinations of these. All of the dilutions were considered to be at levels below the point at which a clas-sical vaccination response could be expected. In fact, the dilutions were tested for presence of viable bacteria and none had any. Obviously, the 30c, 200c, and 1,000c potencies would not likely have even a molecule of nosode matter within it.

Jonas's trial followed every possible protocol one would expect from a rigorous medical experiment. The assignment of mice to control and test groups was random, and every mouse was administered oral prepa-rations through a sterile pipette. The control group was given 70 percent ethanol, and the test group was given the nosode. Dosing occurred 16 times over the period of a month, after which all mice were challenged by a lethal dose of the deadly organism. Afterward, each mouse was given the nosode or the control liquid twice a day for 20 days, or until their death. What were the results? As Jonas reports,

> "Mean time to death for the [nosode]-treated mice was 18.6 days; for controls it was 13.7 days... Overall mortality was 53% in the nosode-treated group and 75% in the matched control group... Therefore, the nosode treatment prevented 22% of deaths... In the control group, exposure to 6,000 CFU (colony forming unit) per animal was required to kill half the animals, whereas in the nosode group exposure to 20,000 CFU per animal was required to produce the same mortality rate. No individual nosode level [potency] disproportionately influenced the overall result." [Jonas, pp. 39–40]. (All results with at least 96% confidence, $p < .04$.)

As part of this trial, Jonas also gave three small groups of mice the standard vaccine for this disease; all survived. Thus, while the nosode definitely afforded a significant level of protection, it was not equal to that of standard vaccination.

Several important points can be made about this rigorous study. First and foremost, it incontrovertibly demonstrates that *potencies beyond Avogadro's number have strong effects beyond that of placebo.* The phenomenon is real. Second, the study demonstrates that homeopathic nosodes represent a potentially lifesaving approach to public health emergencies. Despite the fact that homeopaths do not generally consider nosodes to be the most effective homeopathic prophylaxis against disease (remedies that match an epidemic's symptoms do better — see Chapter 6), the homeopathic literature of the past has many illustrations of the success of this method. For example, as mentioned in the preceding chapter, nosodes were effective in a smallpox outbreak in Iowa in 1902 [Eaton, Traub], and studies in the 1930s and 1940s demonstrated the effectiveness of nosodes in creating immunity to diphtheria [Hoover]. In Jonas's study, a 22% degree of protection was afforded to the mice by taking the nosode. This result alone should be of clinical importance to allopaths and the Center for Disease Control, which do not have an effective vaccine for every disease. If an inexpensive and easily prepared homeopathic nosode could save 22 percent of the people infected with a deadly epidemic, it would certainly be worthwhile. Indeed, as Jonas points out in his paper, this is "especially important as the world becomes increasingly mobile, resistant organisms continue to emerge, and risk of terrorist attacks with biological agents increases." [Jonas, p. 40] In fact, Jonas published this paper in 1999 — long before the September 11, 2001, attacks on the United States. He subsequently testified before Congress in November 2001 about the importance of homeopathy in dealing with the threat of bioterrorism [Jonas01].

THE RANDOMIZED PLACEBO-CONTROLLED TRIAL — THE ONLY PROOF OF EFFECTIVENESS?

Of course, homeopaths know that effects of their remedies are not due to the placebo effect. Lasting cures of chronic disease, not an uncommon occurrence in most homeopathic practices, do not often occur because of "suggestion." If that were true, most of the people who visit homeopaths would have been cured long ago by their allopathic doctors.

Indeed, despite skeptical assertions that homeopathy is beyond the pale of science, homeopaths regard their discipline as extremely scientific — indeed, more scientific than allopathy. After all, rather than using a set of treatments developed in an ad hoc way, homeopaths adhere to a specific law of therapeutics that states exactly which remedies will help to cure a disease. And the basis for application of that law — the effects of remedies on healthy individuals — has always been determined experimentally in the homeopathic proving.

At the same time, however, many homeopaths rankle at using the standard medical trial model — the placebo-controlled double-blind trial — to prove the effectiveness of homeopathy. For one thing, the existence of the Law of Similars makes such trials superfluous. If a medicine has been shown to have specific effects on healthy provers, then its curative effects on the sick are already known. Homeopaths also question the appropriateness of the conventional trial model for homeopathy. The allopathic model usually tests the effects of a single medicine that is given to all participants, regardless of their individual symptoms. In contrast, a fair homeopathic trial must allow for individualized treatment and the use of many possible remedies in different potencies.

The individualized nature of homeopathic treatment has two other features that work against it under the standard trial model. First, and perhaps most important, the success of homeopathic treatment is dependent on the ability of a homeopath to find a correct remedy for a patient. How can a study control for this factor? Practitioner skill is simply not a factor in allopathic studies, since every patient is given the same medicine in the same dose. A second problem is that good homeopathic treatment requires an extensive intake interview. Because of this, a blinded trial must allow a control group to undergo an interview as well. Since the interview process itself can have therapeutic effects, the control group is given an added boost. Indeed, some homeopaths believe that the mere intention of giving a particular remedy to a patient can have some effect in the short term. If this is true, then some form of therapeutic information may be passed to the placebo group as well.

Some medical scientists question the placebo-controlled trial method altogether. If the placebo effect is a therapeutic phenomenon in and of itself, why try to eliminate it? Dimitri Viza, director of the Immunobiology Laboratory at the Facultés de Médecine des Saints-Peres in Paris writes:

> "Today's biomedical science oscillates between rigorous approaches, with rational attitudes, and irrationality or incoherence. Thus, in the era of molecular biology, psychoanalysis thrives and represents a multimillion-dollar annual business, whereas other such 'nonmaterialistic' disciplines as homeopathy, acupuncture, or hypnosis are a priori and uncritically rejected by hard science... But if reason has partially freed us from medieval beliefs, it is now proving to be self-destructive... For when facts are rejected as unreasonable in the name of reason, we are adopting the same superstitious approach to reality as people did in the Middle Ages.
>
> The placebo effect is a perfect illustration of scientific exorcism of a disturbing fact... All efforts are directed not toward studying its

mechanisms, but to subtracting its interference. To satisfy statisticians and referees, constraints have become more stringent and ethics are bent — as are coherence and logic — so that one is justified in wondering whether randomized clinical trials, necessary for producing placebo-free data, are not 'the worst kind of epidemiology,' deliberately ignoring the individual patient's welfare in the name of science...

If, for a number of patients, an inert substance with nil toxicity produces the same beneficial results as a toxic pharmaceutical compound, logic would require that the phenomenon be thoroughly investigated for the patient's benefit, and for its potential to reduce medical cost... In France, for instance, where homeopathic drugs are used by one-third of the population and paid for by national health insurance, their cost represents only one percent of that of conventional drugs. Whether observed clinical improvements are illusory or due to placebo effect, the results satisfy the vast majority of patients and physicians who use these compounds, even if it is shocking for well-thinking scientists to accept that high dilutions of chemicals can display activity, as the homeopathy theory claims. In an era when over-medication threatens the basis of health policies, the rationale for encouraging the fashion for innocuous, low-cost, and yet effective medicines is evident...

Nobody seems to be interested in exploiting homeopathy as a placebo tool, or in funding bona fide research that should prove (or disprove) the underlying theory. Here, again, the attitudes of the proponents and opponents of the hypothesis evoke religious wars, irrationality, and intellectual dishonesty. Yet, several clinical studies suggest genuine effects (K. Linde et al., Lancet, 350:824–5, 1997). But the debate being a passionate one, it will probably never come to a head, every side determined to debunk and ridicule the opponent's position before even considering the evidence." [Viza]

(Copyright ©1998 by The Scientist *LLC, all rights reserved. Reprinted with permission.)*

IT DOES WORK, AND IT WORKS WELL

Despite objections to the standard trial model within the homeopathic community, an increasing number of high-quality randomized placebo-controlled trials of homeopathy are being conducted. One such trial was published by Jennifer Jacobs, MD, and her colleagues in a 1994 issue of *Pediatrics* [Jacobs]. It describes the use of homeopathic remedies for the treatment of acute childhood diarrhea in Nicaragua. This disease was an excellent study target for several reasons. First, severe diarrhea of this kind is an acute process and has a fairly predictable course and suite of symptoms; as a result, the set of likely remedy choices can be determined in advance fairly accurately. While the treatment method in the study was, in fact, individualized (18 different remedies were used and all at a high-dilution of 30c), 60 percent of the children ended up being given one of three remedy choices: *Podophyllum* (made from may apple), *Chamomilla* (made from German chamomile), and *Arsenicum Album* (made from arsenic trioxide).

Another reason why acute childhood diarrhea was an excellent study target is that it is the leading cause of pediatric death worldwide. In developing countries, there are an estimated 1.3 billion cases and 5 million deaths each year among children under age five. One explanation for this high death toll is the fact that the standard recommended treatment — oral rehydration (i.e., administering fluids to the child) — does not really cure the disease. While oral rehydration can sometimes prevent death, it does not decrease the amount of diarrhea nor shorten the duration of the disease. If homeopathic treatment could be shown to be more effective than rehydration, even by a small amount, the positive impact on mortality would be considerable. Moreover, because there is no allopathic medicine that is routinely used for this condition in these countries, standard allopathic treatment would not have to be withheld during the trial. Finally, because acute childhood diarrhea is well understood — for instance, its duration and course is fairly predictable — the impact of homeopathic treatment could easily be measured.

The researchers in this trial took many steps in order to adhere to rigorous scientific procedure. Originally, 92 children were entered into the trial, with 81 completing it satisfactorily. These 81 children ranged from age six months to five years and were randomly assigned to treatment and control groups — 40 in the treatment group and 41 in the control group.

Children were admitted to the study only if they had three or more unformed stools in the previous 24 hours. Severely ill children (Type C dehydration), children who had diarrhea for more than a week, or those who had been given allopathic medicines within the past 48 hours were excluded. All of the children, both control and treatment group, were given oral rehydration therapy during the entire course of the study.

After being weighed, each child underwent a complete homeopathic interview and was assigned a diarrhea severity index score that measured several aspects of their case: amount of vomiting, abdominal pain, temperature, number of unformed stools in the past 24 hours, and level of dehydration. Each child's symptoms were then characterized according to a set of predetermined symptom specifications and entered into a computerized homeopathic expert system that made the final remedy choice. The treating homeopath then prescribed the single remedy that was recommended by the computer system in the 30c potency. Identical looking remedy pellets and placebo pellets were used that had been placed in randomized vials by a pharmacy in the United States. Thus, not even the homeopaths knew which was which. Parents were then instructed to give their child one pellet of medication after each unformed stool and to note their actions on a treatment card. Follow-up home visits were made each day for the next five days by community health workers, who examined both the child and the treatment cards. After five days, each child was reweighed.

What were the results? Although the control and treatment groups had no significant pretrial differences in age, height, weight, or severity of disease, homeopathic treatment did make a significant difference in the outcome for the two groups (all results are with 95% confidence, $p < .05$). Table 2 shows that three important aspects of the disease course were reduced by one day: the number of days until there were less than three unformed stools on two consecutive days; the number of days until there was 50 percent improvement; and the number of days until the first formed stool appeared. This is a significant improvement for this disease, since its usual duration is only five or six days to begin with. A guarantee of one less day of diarrhea could have a significant impact on childhood mortality all over the world.

The stool of the children in the Jacobs study was also tested for the presence of certain bacteria and viruses. Interestingly, homeopathic treatment had its most dramatic effects on children who tested positive for these pathogens. I am sure that many skeptics will not believe that homeopathy could have a measurable impact on a disease where bacteria and viruses are measurable and present. But this study provides evidence quite to the contrary. In fact, Dr. Jacobs went on to successfully replicate her diarrhea study with a second trial conducted in Nepal [Jacobs00].

Table 2:

Reproduced by permission of Pediatrics, Volume 93, Page 722, Table 5, Copyright 1994.

	Homeopathic Treatment	*Control*
Days to < 3 unformed stools on 2 consecutive days		
Median	*2.5*	*4.0*
Mean	*3.0*	*3.8*
Days to 50% improvement		
Median	*1.0*	*2.0*
Mean	*1.9*	*2.7*
Days to first formed stool		
Median	*3.0*	*5.5*
Mean	*3.6*	*4.4*
Weight/Height Percentile Change		
Median	*6.0*	*1.0*
Mean	*4.6*	*2.8*

Now let's look at another clinical trial — this time with animal subjects. In 1999, a German study on commercially farmed pigs was published that has the potential, like the diarrhea study, to have a great impact on world health [Albrecht]. In modern livestock farms, it is routine to administer low levels of antibiotics in order to prevent rampant disease. This study compared outcomes for four randomly assigned groups of pigs that were administered either placebo, homeopathic treatment (in this case, a combination of five different remedies in various potencies), a standard blend of antibiotics and other allopathic drugs in a routine low prophylactic dose, and a standard blend of allopathic drugs in a high therapeutic dose. There were 1440 pigs involved in the study, which took place at an intensive livestock farm in northern Germany. The primary outcome measured was the incidence of respiratory disease, which normally affects 24 percent to 69 percent of pigs on such farms.

The results of this study were startling: *homeopathic treatment was far superior to prophylactic doses of antibiotics in preventing respiratory disease.* Prophylactic allopathic treatment made it only 11 percent less likely (than placebo) that the pigs would become sick. But homeopathic remedies made it *40 percent* less likely. When the allopathic drugs were raised to therapeutic levels, it became 70 percent less likely that the pigs would become diseased. Now, it is clearly impossible to keep farmed animals medicated at high levels of antibiotics all of the time. Even at lower prophylactic levels, the entrance of these drugs into the food chain has become a societal health problem. This study showed that homeopathy provides a much safer and more effective solution than prophylactic antibiotics.

I believe it is animal studies like this one that provide the most compelling proof of the effectiveness of homeopathy. Can anyone seriously believe that pigs taking remedies in their feeding trough are getting well because of the placebo effect? Indeed, the improvement in this case was 40 percent better than placebo — and 29 percent better than standard allopathic treatment. Yet has this information been heeded? Or have the results of the Jacobs study been taken seriously and made an impact on the treatment of childhood diarrhea around the world? Unfortunately, the answer is: no.

There are a great many other studies out there — too numerous to be discussed in detail here. The greatest percentage of them are being published in Europe, where homeopathy is more accepted than it is in the United States. Another exciting development in recent years is the initiation of several large-scale multicenter studies in Europe that include thousands of patients [GermanStudies]. A few short summaries of some notable trial results are presented below. For those interested in finding out more, two books that are easily accessible to an American audience are the aforementioned book by Jonas and Jacobs [Jonas&Jacobs] and a more recent book by Bill Gray, MD [Gray]. Another book that reviews trials, but focuses primarily on scientific explanations for how homeopathic remedies might work, was published by two Italian physicians, Paolo Bellavite, MD, and Andrea Signorini, MD [Bellavite].

Rheumatoid Arthritis Study, 1980
Gibson and colleagues in Glasgow, Scotland, performed a double-blind controlled trial of homeopathic treatment in rheumatoid arthritis patients with careful assessment of progress. There were only 23 patients in each group. Both had full homeopathic interviews but the control group got placebo instead of remedy. Nineteen showed improvement in the treatment group compared to five in the placebo group. [Gibson]

Allergy Study, 1994
David Reilly, MD, and colleagues in Glasgow performed a double-blind controlled trial of a 30c potency of house dust mite, given to dust-allergy sufferers. In the homeopathic group 77 percent showed an improvement compared to only 33 percent showing an improvement with placebo. The study was supervised by a consulting respiratory physician who recruited the patients for the study. [Reilly94]

Trials of Oscillococcinum for Flu, 1989 and 1998
Oscillococcinum is a commercial flu remedy marketed by Boiron, a French homeopathic pharmacy. The remedy is made from duck's liver in the 200c potency. A study in the April 1998 issue of the *British Homeopathic Journal* reported that 17.4 percent of those taking

Oscillococcinum were symptom-free the day after treatment began, compared to 6.6 percent of those taking placebo. In a similar study published in the March 1989 issue of the *British Journal of Clinical Pharmacology*, 24.6 percent of those with mild to moderate symptoms had recovered by the second day, compared to 11.9 percent of those taking placebo. [Ferley, Papp]

Aconite for Postoperative Pain and Agitation in Children, 1990

Pain and agitation are common postoperative symptoms. Fifty children with symptoms similar to those of *Aconite* (made from monkshood, a flower) — violent, sudden, and intense anguish — were given either placebo or Aconite in this double-blind study. The Aconite had good results in 95 percent of the cases. The authors concluded, "This remedy has a place in the recovery-room and should be in every physician's emergency case." [Alibeu]

Allergy Study, 2000

In the summer of 2000, another allergy study by Reilly and his colleagues at the Glasgow Homeopathic Hospital was published in the *British Medical Journal*. Fifty patients were treated with a homeopathic preparation or with placebo, and were measured daily for nasal air flow. Those on homeopathic treatment had 28 percent improved nasal air flow over the course of four weeks, compared with just 3 percent improvement in the placebo group. [Reilly00]

Recovery in Alcoholics and Drug Addicts, 2000

In this study, 703 alcoholics and drug addicts in a large detox center were randomized into three groups. One group received a single dose of an individually prescribed homeopathic remedy, another received a single dose of placebo, and the third group received nothing. All other medications and modalities utilized were identical for the three groups. The study found that the placebo and control groups had limited and similar results — 68 percent of the placebo group had relapsed after 18 months, and 72 percent of the control group. In contrast, only 32 percent of the homeopathic group relapsed. The homeopathic group also had highly significant improvement in various measurements of physical and psychological health. Interestingly, those who received homeopathic treatment also experienced various "cleansing" reactions in the first three days after treatment, such as nasal discharge and skin rashes. [Garcia-Swain]

Otitis Media Study, 2001

Jennifer Jacobs, MD, and her colleagues have recently published another trial in the *Pediatric Infectious Disease Journal* [Jacobs01]. It studied the homeopathic treatment of acute otitis media (ear infection) in children, the most common illness for which pediatricians are consulted. An estimated 55 percent of children in the United States receive antibiotics for this ailment by the time they are one year old. The 75 children in this randomized placebo-controlled study ranged in age from 18 months to six years old and were experiencing middle ear infection for no more than 36 hours. Only eight homeopathic remedies were allowed for use, making the potential outcome slightly less favorable for homeopathic treatment. What was the result?

There was a significant decrease in symptoms at 24 and 64 hours after treatment in the group treated homeopathically. Overall, there were 19.9 percent more treatment failures in the placebo group than in the homeopathic group. Since an estimated 70 percent to 90 percent of otitis media cases resolve on their own anyway, this amount of difference between the two groups is striking. Although parents were permitted to administer analgesics if they felt it were necessary, children in the homeopathic group were given such drugs half as often as children in the placebo group. This study could be a potential breakthrough in the management of pediatric otitis media, since pediatricians are currently trying to forego antibiotic treatment unless it is really necessary. Indeed, homeopathic treatment can provide pediatricians with a proven technique that could help them to succeed.

The Indian Experience

The most extensive homeopathic research trials today are probably taking place in India, where homeopathy is a fully accepted medical system, with its own medical schools and hospitals. Many Indian homeopaths operate large clinics where they see hundreds of patients each day. Unlike the quiet office environments in which most Western homeopaths practice, a typical Indian clinic is crowded with hundreds of people waiting in line with their families. Intake interviews are conducted by resident homeopaths who are studying and training there. When a patient finally speaks to the chief homeopath, it is usually in a room crowded with other people who have been waiting in line for hours. It is not unusual for the patient and family members to shout out the most personal symptoms during this brief 5- or 10-minute interview. After such a long wait, there is no time for beating around the bush!

Because of this environment, Indian homeopaths are able to see vastly more patients than their European and American counterparts. They are also able to treat a much wider range of diseases: tuberculosis, leprosy, malaria, cancer — anything you can imagine. Because of the clinical freedom that Indian homeopaths have, some fascinating large-scale research studies have been possible. For example, they have been able to systematically experiment with different potencies, remedies, and dosing regimens for specific ailments.

One exciting development in recent years is the success some Indian homeopaths have been having in treating HIV disease. In April 1999, the *British Homeopathic Journal* published a study by homeopaths from the Central Council for Research in Homeopathy in New Delhi, and the Regional Research Institute for Homeopathy in Bombay [Rastogi]. This randomized double-blind placebo-controlled trial assessed the effect of homeopathic treatment on patients with CD4-positive T-lymphocytes, a laboratory indicator of the severity of HIV progression. One hundred HIV-positive individuals between the ages of 18 and 50 took part in the six-month study, with 50 cases at stage II (asymptomatic) HIV and 50 cases at stage III. A single individualized homeopathic remedy was prescribed in each case. The main outcome measure of the study was the patients' CD4-positive T-lymphocyte counts.

The net result of this study was that, in the more severely sick group (stage III), there was a statistically significant improvement for the homeopathically treated group, but no significant change for the place-bo group. After the initial six-month trial, the 100 participants were joined by an additional 550 HIV-infected patients, who were then all treated. The May 1999 issue of *Homeopathy Today* reported on the results. According to a press release by the Indian government, "After a period of 3 to 16 months, many patients gave non-reactive response to ELISA and some gave negative response to Western blot test [both standard tests for HIV] indicating effectiveness of the therapy" [India]. As a result, the Indian government has established new homeopathic research laborato-ries for HIV research.

META-ANALYSIS

One of the primary complaints lodged by skeptics of homeopathy is that homeopathic trials have not been sufficiently replicated. While it is true that few homeopathic studies have yet to be precisely repeated by inde-pendent teams, the same can be said of many allopathic medical trials. For this reason, a statistical method has been developed that enables researchers to overcome this problem: *meta-analysis*. In a meta-analysis, several diverse experiments that study the same phenomenon can be combined and analyzed collectively. This enables researchers to deter-mine whether the effects measured do indeed demonstrate that a phe-nomenon is replicable.

Some of you may be familiar with the allopathic research finding that taking a daily aspirin can help to prevent heart attacks. This discov-ery was the result of a meta-analysis. The study, first reported in the *British Medical Journal* in 1988, was widely acclaimed as a medical break-through and has been used as a model for medical meta-analysis since that time. Twenty-five different studies that examined the effects of aspirin on reducing heart attacks were combined. Although only five studies were individually successful, when the results were combined, there was no doubt left about aspirin's benefits.

> "Considered individually, the majority (80 percent) of the studies are 'failures'... A reviewer who was skeptical of aspirin's ability to reduce heart attacks might examine these individual studies and go away unimpressed, confident that there was no evidence that aspirin has any clear therapeutic value... When the results of all the studies are *combined*, the overall result... clearly excludes chance. Thus, even though the effect is uncertain when considered in individual experiments, it was widely advertised (and rightly so) that taking aspirin really does make a significant difference." [Radin, pp. 55–56]

Because existing studies on homeopathy are quite diverse — they use a variety of different remedies on a wide range of conditions — meta-analysis is a perfect way to test whether or not the effects of homeopathic remedies are real or are merely due to the placebo effect. Two such meta-analyses have already been conducted: one published in 1991 [Kleijnen] and another published in 1997 [Linde]. Both of these studies demonstrated that the effects of homeopathic remedies dramatically exceed those of placebo. In fact, the latter study, published by Klaus Linde and his colleagues in the highly respected British medical journal, *The Lancet*, found that homeopathy, on average, performed nearly 2½ times better (was nearly 250 percent more effective) than placebo. This astounding result would be enviable in most allopathic trials. For example, in the aspirin study mentioned above, aspirin was only 75 percent better than placebo. Let's take a closer look at what the researchers of the Linde study found.

Beginning with an initial set of 186 homeopathic trials, Linde and his colleagues narrowed their focus to 89 trials that met prespecified criteria. These included: the use of a placebo control group (119 met this criterion); a focus on the treatment of a specific clinical condition in humans (rather than a tissue study, animal study, or a study conducted on healthy subjects such as a proving); the use of random assignment of the test subjects to the placebo or homeopathic group, or the use of double-blinding; publication in scholarly form; sufficient information for data extraction purposes; and exclusion of single-case studies.

Out of the 89 selected homeopathic studies, 13 used classical homeopathy (individualized treatment according to the totality of symptoms), 49 used "clinical" homeopathy (the targeted ailment was treated with a predetermined remedy rather than according to the patient's individual symptoms), 20 used polypharmacy (combination remedies), and 7 used isopathy. In addition, out of the 89 studies, 31 used high-potency remedies in excess of 12c (dilutions beyond Avogadro's number) and 51 used potencies in excess of 5c (with estimated molar concentrations lower than 10^{-13}). The average study was conducted on 118 patients, with a median of 60 patients per study. When study quality was measured (two separate measures were used), 26 were deemed very high in quality and 40 were of good quality.

Table 3 provides some of the pooled results of the meta-analysis. All results are provided in terms of an odds ratio that measures the relative superiority of the homeopathic remedy in comparison to placebo. Thus, a measure of 1 means that placebo and the homeopathic remedy were equal in effect. A result that is less than 1 means that placebo was superior to homeopathy. A measure of x, where x is greater than 1, means that homeopathy was approximately x times as effective as the placebo group. All of the results were deemed accurate with 95 percent confidence [Linde].

As shown in the table, the results for all of the 89 studies combined yields an odds ratio of 2.45. Thus, overall, homeopathic remedies were found to be about 2.45 times as effective as (245 percent better than) placebo. If just the 26 high-quality studies are included, homeopathy was still much more effective, with an odds ratio of 1.66 — i.e., around 66 percent better than placebo. Interestingly, the studies that had good patient follow-up did much better, with a ratio of 3.18. The success of these longer-term trials provides further proof that homeopathic effects are not due to placebo; placebo effects are notoriously short-lived, whereas homeopathic effects are not.

Table 3:

Reprinted with permission from Elsevier Science *(The Lancet, 1997, Volume 250, Page 838).*

	Number of Studies	Odds Ratio (95% confidence interval)
All Studies	89	*2.45 (2.05, 2.93)*
High-Quality	26	*1.66 (1.33, 2.08)*
Adequate Concealment	34	*1.93 (1.51, 2.47)*
Double-Blinding Stated	81	*2.17 (1.83, 2.57)*
Adequate Followup	28	*3.18 (2.14, 4.73)*
MEDLINE Listed	23	*1.70 (1.31, 2.20)*
Corrected For Possible Bias	89	*1.78 (1.03, 3.10)*
Worst Case Scenario	5	*1.97 (1.04, 3.75)*
High Potencies	31	*2.66 (1.83, 3.87)*
High/Medium Potencies	51	*2.77 (2.09, 3.67)*
Classical	13	*2.91 (1.57, 5.37)*
Clinical	49	*2.00 (1.60, 2.51)*
Isopathy	7	*5.04 (2.24, 11.32)*
Polypharmacy	20	*2.94 (2.12, 3.08)*

The Linde study also tried to examine the credibility factor in their analysis. First, they tried to account for any possible publication bias in favor of homeopathy, with the assumption that studies may have under-reported bad results. Even so, the odds ratio remained at 1.78. In fact, it was estimated that there would have to be 923 missing trials of average size (118 patients) with results demonstrating an effect equal to placebo in order to dismiss the results in favor of homeopathy. Since there are probably not 923 homeopathic trials in existence, this possibility seems very unlikely. The meta-analysis authors even identified a worst-case scenario — grouping together only those studies that were most likely not to favor homeopathy — i.e., those studies that were of high quality, published on MEDLINE, and that used medium or high dilutions. Even so, this small group of five studies got a rating of 1.97.

Another fascinating result of the Linde study was its assessment of the effects of potency and homeopathic methodology on the results obtained. As it turns out, the high- and high/medium-potency studies did better than the overall result, with the high-potency studies yielding an odds ratio of 2.66 and the high/medium-potency studies yielding a score of 2.77. As far as methodology, isopathy got the highest score of 5.04 (i.e., five times better than placebo), though with a wide confidence range since there were only seven such studies. Classical homeopathy and polypharmacy did about equally well, with scores of 2.91 and 2.94 respectively. Clinical (nonindividualized) homeopathy, which was used in the majority of the studies, did the worst, with a score of 2.00.

Not surprisingly, many objections to the Linde study were lodged in the allopathic literature. Many people were quick to cite the following quote from the paper: "There is insufficient evidence from these studies that any *single type of homeopathic treatment* is clearly effective in any *one clinical condition*" [Linde, p.839] (italic emphasis is my own). In fact, most reports about this study in the allopathic literature quoted this sentence alone — *and eliminated any discussion of the 2.45 odds-ratio result*. Thus, they cleverly omitted the primary result of the study — that homeopathy's effectiveness is *not* due to placebo.

Of course, this quote from the study is completely true. There was not sufficient evidence to state that any *one* particular type of homeopathic treatment was clearly effective in any *one* clinical condition. That is because the 89 studies collectively utilized four different kinds of homeopathic treatment, and administered a myriad of different remedies and potencies for many different kinds of conditions. The purpose of this study was not to test whether a particular treatment was effective for a particular condition. Rather, its goal was to find out whether the overall effects of homeopathy were better than those of placebo. And it very clearly did demonstrate that fact.

The Linde study also brought out the debunkers, who were quick to question the quality of the homeopathic trials that were included, despite that fact that trial quality was measured as part of the meta-analysis. Such skepticism is, unfortunately, quite typical, and it also reflects a severe double standard. In a 1998 *Lancet* article written by Canadian epidemiologist David Moher and his colleagues, 127 allopathic trials conducted between 1960 and 1995 were reviewed. They found that results reported by allopathic trials were often exaggerated or flawed. For instance, treatment results were exaggerated by 30 percent to 50 percent because of experimental irregularities such as failing to report when patients dropped out of a trial. In some cases, previously touted results were found to have no validity at all. For example, studies that claimed that the anticoagulant drug LMW heparin reduces deaths from blood clots by 47 percent were found, upon closer inspection, to provide no evidence at all that the drug prevents death [Moher].

Indeed, more and more scandals in the allopathic medical research community have emerged in recent years. An investigation reported in the *New York Times*, for example, found that many highly lucrative allopathic drug trials are being conducted by private doctors on their patients in unethical and sloppy ways [NYTimes]. There has also been increasing evidence that research results, and even the policies of the FDA, suffer from egregious conflicts of interest due to the influence of pharmaceutical companies [Rosenstock, USAToday]. In contrast, those who conduct homeopathic drug trials are painfully aware of the scrutiny their work will be subjected to. Despite meager funding for their trials, homeopathic researchers try to be even more disciplined, ethical, and scientific than many of their allopathic peers.

THE MESSAGE AND THE MEDIUM

So the effects of homeopathic remedies are real and beneficial. But how do they work? The truth is, so far, no one really knows for sure. There are many models and theories that homeopaths have developed over the years, but modern science is simply not yet able to determine exactly how homeopathic ultradilutions do their job. Nor is there any real understanding of why treatment according to the Law of Similars yields such effective cures. Nevertheless, there are some glimmers of illumination beginning to appear in the realms of physical chemistry and biophysics, and in the application of ideas from mathematical complexity and chaos theory to systems of the human body. This section will consider some of these results and their implications.

Let's begin by looking at homeopathy in terms of complexity and chaos theory. An excellent text on this subject is *The Emerging Science of Homeopathy: Complexity, Biodynamics, and Nanopharmacology,* by Bellavite and Signorini [Bellavite]. Another older, yet still quite excellent text is *Scientific Foundations of Homeopathy,* by G. Resch and V. Gutmann [Resch]. As Bellavite and Signorini point out, the human body is undeniably a system that is complex in a formal sense. Complex systems are inherently unpredictable and chaotic, even if they can also manifest predictable phenomena. Indeed, even a simple closed system can become chaotic if it is sensitive to conditions from outside the system. For example, the behavior of a large set of billiard balls hit by an initial collision can quickly become chaotic. Another well-known illustration of this phenomenon is the *butterfly effect,* "the principle embodied in... the dictum that the flapping of butterfly's wings in Brazil may trigger off or stop in its tracks, a tornado in Texas." [Bellavite, p. 161]

Despite their unpredictable nature, chaotic systems can also manifest order when viewed in the large. For example, they can manifest *fractal properties,* wherein similar forms or structures emerge when the system is viewed at varying levels of detail. A typical illustration of fractals is the kinds of patterns that can be found in flower petals. The stable effects and patterns found in otherwise chaotic systems are created by *attractors* — factors that somehow pull a system toward structure rather than chaos.

Bellative and Signorini surmise that disease occurs in complex human systems because they are influenced by *pathological attractors*; in homeopathic terms, because the vital force becomes distorted by an exciting cause [Bellavite, p. 175]. Sometimes the net effect of these pathological attractors is to render a normally chaotic system overly stable and rigid, and therefore unable to adapt [Bellavite, p. 177]. This is analogous to homeopathy's notion of the vital force becoming stuck in a disease posture — i.e., it can no longer reachieve balance. Bellavite and Signorini also suggest that when a body becomes chronically diseased, it has actually become *habituated* to a pathological attractor. Because it has gotten used to this disease signal, it no longer responds with an appropriate defense.

Bellavite and Signorini go on to suggest that homeopathy's dilute doses have such profound effects because complex systems are inherently sensitive to small precise signals.

> "A system which obeys the laws of complexity does not always behave in a linear manner; i.e., the effects are not always proportional to the doses of a given factor which modifies the equilibrium... In the behavior of complex systems, the quality of information is far more important than the quantity... When a system is in a state of dys–equilibrium controlled by many factors, i.e., when it presents a behavior pattern characterized by complexity and chaos, a *small amount* of energy should be enough to make it shift one way or another. The nearer one is to the bifurcation point, and the greater the freedom of choice, the lower will be the energy needed to shift the system in one direction or another." [Bellavite, pp.187, 190, 285]

According to this argument, homeopathic remedies function as *high-quality attractors* that precisely stimulate necessary changes in the body's complex systems. The quality of a remedy's signal derives from the fact it is chosen to closely match the symptoms of a patient's disease state. In other words, because it is homeopathic to a patient's disease, a remedy can provide a signal that will have just the right effect.

So how exactly do remedies transmit their information to the body? This is where explorations into the nature of water and high dilutions come into play. Although research in this area is still quite preliminary, there are some interesting hints and clues to be found. For example, consider the work of Vittorio Elia, PhD, a professor on the Faculty of

Science in physical chemistry at the University of Naples, who has been specializing in the microcalorimetry of water solutions since 1973. His recent work has demonstrated that measurable excess heat (calories) can be found in succussed ultradilutions and that this heat is retained indefinitely over time. In about 92 percent of the cases studied by Elia, it was shown that successive dilution and succussion permanently altered the physical-chemical properties of solvent water [Elia].

Another new area of study, *cluster physics*, focuses on aggregates of small, finite numbers of atoms or molecules called clusters. Clusters are interesting because their behavior can range from quantum-size effects (in the smallest clusters) to the more stable properties of solids. One sub-area of cluster physics focuses on water clusters. It has been well known for a number of years that water molecules can form stable structures. Since the water molecule is polarized (one side is more positive and other side is more negative), bonds can form between the hydrogen and oxygen atoms of neighboring water molecules to form clusters. The existence of "unprotonated" water cluster ions in large water clusters has been reported since the 1980s [Shinohara]. The stability of water clusters is enhanced by the inclusion of atomic or molecular gases which cause the water molecules to organize cavity-like clusters around them [Sloan, Filipponi]. The precise structure of cluster ions was first determined in 1998 [Jongma].

How are these clusters formed in the lab? One laboratory in Sweden utilizes an apparatus that shoots a gas, under high pressure, into a vacuum. "The resulting... expansion cools the gas, and partial condensation occurs. Clusters are produced as a molecular beam, and un-clustered atoms are removed by large turbo pumps. The size of the clusters is distributed around a mean value, which may be altered by variation of expansion pressure, nozzle diameter, and temperature." [Uppsala] Could homeopathic potentization, and in particular, succussion, achieve a similar effect? Do ultradilutions contain clustered water? As homeopath and former chemical engineer Brian Connelly points out, succussion causes *cavitation*, the creation of partial vacuums in a liquid [Connelly]. This cavitation is accompanied by heat and kinetic energy that provides a unique chemical environment within the liquid (as was shown by Elia). It is thus within the realm of possibility that succussion could enable the creation of stable water clusters.

Recent studies have also shown that alcohol can form clusters. These clusters are ring-shaped, in contrast to the linear stretches that form in water clusters [Provencal]. The structure of alcohol clusters might explain why the use of a mixture of water and alcohol for homeopathic potentization helps to stabilize the properties of homeopathic potencies. Indeed, as I will describe next, recent biomedical research with ultradilutions has affirmed the importance of alcohol's role in potentization.

Jacques Benveniste, MD, a French allopath, is a world-famous medical researcher who discovered Platelet Activating Factor in 1970. Unfortunately, his career was set upon a rocky course after he published his first paper on ultradilutions. It all began when a colleague encouraged him to make a study of the phenomenon. Much to his own surprise, Benveniste found that ultradilutions in excess of Avogadro's number could consistently have the same effects as the original solute substance — but only if the dilution process was accompanied by vigorous agitation of the solution (i.e., succussion).

Benveniste's landmark paper in *Nature*, "Human Basophil Degranulation Triggered by Very Dilute Antiserum Against IgE" [Benveniste88], described how antibodies of immunoglobulin E (anti-IgE) could degranulate human basophils (a standard response) even when the anti-IgE was diluted and succussed up to 10^{120} — far in excess of Avogadro's number at 10^{23}. This activity was established under stringent experimental conditions, including double-blinding, and was carried out across six laboratories in four countries. As a control, Benveniste also created an ultradilution of a different kind of antibody, anti-IgG; but the potentized anti-IgG did *not* yield the same response. When he then created ultradilutions of other substances known to have similar effects on the basophils as anti-IgE, they yielded the appropriate response. Thus, Benveniste's experiments demonstrated that *the potentization process maintains the specific action of a substance, even after the original molecules are absent.* In fact, Benveniste's high potencies were actually tested for the presence of the original substance, and it was absent.

Since the 1988 publication of his discovery, Benveniste's work has been subjected to unending controversy and derision by skeptics. Eventually, he lost his research funding and laboratory, and he was forced to continue work on his own. But he did continue.

In 2001, Benveniste was finally vindicated. A team of scientists led by once-skeptical Professor Madeleine Ennis of Queen's University Belfast obtained results that seem to back up Benveniste's original work [Ennis]. Ennis's team did not replicate Benveniste's work precisely; instead, they tested the ability of ultradilutions of histamine to *inhibit* the degranulation of basophils caused by anti-IgE. Much to their own amazement, however, these succussed ultradilutions did have the appropriate effect. As reported in the March 15, 2001 issue of the *Guardian Weekly* [Milgrom], Ennis and her collaborators went to great lengths to eliminate the chance of bias in their study. Four different laboratories were involved, three of which prepared the solutions and controls and were not involved in any other way. The contents of all solutions and controls was blinded and an independent researcher collated the final data. Ennis even developed a method for collecting data that could be completely automated. Nevertheless, the results held.

Ironically, Benveniste, like most of the scientists working on ultradilutions, has no interest in homeopathy; he is a confirmed allopath. Benveniste's main interest in ultradilutions is their use as a vehicle for the delivery of allopathic medicines. But in the course of his work, he has managed to rediscover many properties of ultradilutions that homeopaths have known for nearly two hundred years. These include the following:

- The agitation (succussion) step is necessary to create effective ultradilutions. Experiments with simple dilutions (created without succussion) did not yield the same response.

- Ultradilutions tend to yield better responses at certain potencies, exhibiting a kind of periodic dose-effect curve. This may explain why homeopaths tend to use specific centesimal potencies — for example, 6c, 12c, 18c, 24c, 30c, 200c, 1,000c, etc.

- Exposure to severe heat degrades the effects of ultradilutions. Benveniste believes this cutoff to be 70° C or 158° F. Interestingly, both Benveniste and homeopaths have found that succussion of degraded remedies tends to restore some of their effects.

- The most effective diluent for creating ultradilutions is a mixture of alcohol and water. This was also recommended by Hahnemann, and seems to stabilize the information in a dilution so that it can last for years. Every homeopath knows that properly stored remedies can retain their effects indefinitely. I personally know people who have successfully utilized remedy kits that belonged to homeopaths of the 1800s.

Naturally, when Benveniste came upon these properties of ultradilutions, he wondered how they could be acting. Today, he surmises that the potentization process conveys into a solution an electromagnetic signal that is specific to the substance being potentized. In fact, he believes that it is just this kind of electromagnetic signal, conveyed in water, that is the key to how information is carried within biological organisms in general. In other words, when it comes to biological systems, *the message is energetic, and the medium is water.*

Of course, currently accepted doctrine in biochemistry dictates that molecules must be in contact with one another to have effects. But, as Benveniste points out, the successful action of allopathic drugs on the human body seems to disprove this. The molecules of ingested drugs have physical contact with their targets only through random chance; their statistical effectiveness should be fairly low if direct molecular contact was absolutely necessary. In contrast, the electromagnetic signal of a substance can be carried effectively throughout the body (via water) without a substance coming into contact with target cells. Benveniste insists that this theory does not violate any current biological or physical principles. It is well known that molecules emit specific frequencies and that all biological interactions occur in water, which makes up 70 percent to 80 percent of the human body. Indeed, quantum electrodynamics allows for long-range electromagnetic fields to be transmitted in water in just this way.

Benveniste has tested his electromagnetic signaling theory and has come up with even more controversial results. In a 1997 issue of the *Journal on Clinical Immunology* [Benveniste97], he reported that he was able to digitally transmit the electromagnetic signal of an ultradilution of a specific antigen. He did this by first passing a noise signal through an ultradilution and digitally recording the result. He then sent this digitized signal via E-mail from France to Chicago, where it was replayed into water. The resulting water was able to have the expected antigen-specific effects on isolated guinea pig hearts in a Chicago laboratory.

This astounding experiment was conducted under blind conditions in stringent laboratory settings. If the results are to be believed, the consequences are nothing short of mind-boggling. The ability to digitize and electronically transmit biological effects could open up whole new realms of application in medicine. Drugs (both allopathic and homeopathic) could be potentized, digitized, and distributed at essentially zero cost over the Internet. Indeed, any biological or chemical product could be digitized and transmitted in this way.

One interesting characteristic of Benveniste's work is that the digitized ultradilution signals don't have to be understood or decoded into order to be transmitted and used. This "black box" property of homeopathic ultradilutions may, in fact, be one of the greatest strengths of homeopathy. A disease doesn't have to be deciphered or reduced to a biological mechanism in order to be treated. A body's symptoms are its response to a disease signal, and the homeopathic remedy that can cure those symptoms will simply be the one that creates a similar signal. It doesn't matter what's inside the homeopathic black box — as long as the signal pattern of a disease and the signal pattern of a remedy match, the remedy will cure the disease.

Of course, there is much more to be explored. Do remedies cause detectable electromagnetic effects on the body? Is electromagnetism all there is to it? Are there other energy fields at work? These are all questions for future research.

HOMEOPATHIC MODELS OF REMEDY ACTION

Naturally, homeopaths have also been trying to understand how remedies might be acting — long before modern research studies were possible. Most of the models of remedy action that have been developed by homeopaths are based on the assumption that an energetic or nonmaterial force underlies the physical structure of the body and guides its functioning. Homeopathic remedies are considered to operate directly on this unseen body energy — the dynamis or vital force.

Homeopathy's conception of the vital force can be compared to Chinese medicine's *qi* or Indian medicine's *prana.* These Eastern medical disciplines, like homeopathy, view the energy body as primary and the physical body as secondary. For example, a cancerous tumor is seen as the end result of a disease process; the root cause of the cancer lies within the vital force. For this reason, cutting out, irradiating, or poisoning a tumor will not remove a patient's innate tendency to develop cancer. This susceptibility to cancer can only be cured by repairing the vital force.

The homeopathic notion of the vital force sprang from a philosophy called *vitalism* that was popular in Europe and America during the 1800s. Vitalism is based on Aristotle's belief that a nonmaterial soul exists within all living things, and that this soul is the force that organizes the body's activity and gives it directedness and purpose. Modern-day biologist Rupert Sheldrake's theory of *morphic resonance* is a kind of evolutionary form of vitalism. He hypothesizes that a nonmaterial force purposefully links all members of a species together. This morphic field allows the behavioral memories and habits of a species to be inherited and to evolve. Sheldrake writes:

> "Whereas mechanists maintained that living organisms are... machines, vitalists argued that they are truly alive... Vitalists thought that... non-material vital factors organized the bodies and behavior of living organisms in a holistic and purposive manner, drawing organisms towards a realization of their potential forms and ways of behaving, and that when organisms die, the vital factors disappear from them." [Sheldrake, p. 69]

Hahnemann's belief in the existence of the vital force grew as he began to achieve successful cures with very high dilutions. He knew that high-potency remedies were not likely to be acting materially, so he reasoned that their action must be in some other unseen realm — a place where disease truly begins and where true cure must therefore take place. He wrote:

> "When a person falls ill, it is initially only this spirit-like, autonomic life force (life principle), everywhere present in the organism, that is mistuned through the dynamic [i.e., energetic] influence of a morbific agent inimical to life. Only the life principle, mistuned to such abnormality, can impart to the organism the adverse sensations and induce in the organism the irregular functions that we call disease...
>
> Therefore disease is not what allopaths believe it to be. Disease is not to be considered as an inwardly hidden wesen [entity] separate from the living whole, from the organism and its enlivening dynamis, even if it is thought to be very subtle. Such an absurdity could only arise in brains of a materialistic stamp. It is this absurdity that has for thousands of years given to the hitherto system of medicine all those ruinous directions that have fashioned it into a truly calamitous art...
>
> Our life force, as spirit-like dynamis, cannot be seized and affected... other than in a spirit-like, dynamic way. In like manner, the only way the medical-art practitioner can remove such morbid mistunements (the diseases) from the dynamis is by the spirit-like tunement-altering energies of the serviceable medicines acting upon our spirit-like life force... Curative medicines can reestablish health and life's harmony only through dynamic action on the life principle." [Hahnemann, Aphorisms 11, 13, 16]

In this last section, Hahnemann makes reference to the fact that the diseased vital force is "mistuned." It is then "retuned" by the medicinal energy of the remedies. Notice the similarity of this reasoning to that of Bellavite and Signorini's complexity-based model. The body is "mistuned" by a pathological attractor; it is "retuned" by the positive signal provided by a remedy. Hahnemann's vibrational analogy is also similar to Vithoulkas's notion of energetic resonance; in particular, the body's energetic resonance or vibration determines its susceptibility to certain diseases and its cure by certain remedies [Vithoulkas]. Somehow, possibly through a signature embedded in water, the remedies communicate energetically with the energy of the vital force and set it right again. But how? Below are four candidate theories that have been put forth in homeopathic circles.

1. Action-Counteraction

The notion of action and counteraction (reaction) is fundamental in physics — "for each action there is an equal and opposite reaction." This same idea can be used to explain the operation of the vital force. In particular, the healing of the vital force is seen as a counteraction to the stimulus provided by a remedy.

There is much support for this action-counteraction model in the natural responses of the physical body. For example, if you drink a lot of coffee to wake you up, you may eventually rebound and become very tired. Or, if you become energized by eating a lot of sugar, eventually you may react with a sugar "low." The physical body possesses a great number of mechanisms that operate in this way in order to balance and regulate reactions to physiological extremes. Without these regulating mechanisms, which control body temperature, blood content, blood pressure, and more, we would quickly die.

Homeopaths have also seen evidence for the action-counteraction model during provings. For example, when a prover takes a remedy that creates diarrhea symptoms, this diarrhea is sometimes followed by constipation. These action-counteraction responses are called the *primary* and *secondary* responses to a remedy. Hahnemann wrote:

"Each medicine alters the tuning of the life force... and arouses a certain alteration of a person's condition for a longer or shorter time. This
is termed the *initial action*. While the initial action is a product of both
the medicinal energy and the life force, it belongs more to the impinging potence [of the medicine]. Our life force strives to oppose this
impinging action with its own energy. This back-action belongs to our
sustentive power of life and is an automatic function of it, called the
after-action or *counter-action*." [Hahnemann, Aphorism 63]

One way of thinking about the body's action-counteraction reactions is in terms of a pendulum. The body prefers to be in a state where
the pendulum is at its lowest center point — i.e., in a stable steady state.
If the pendulum gets pushed in one direction or another, it will respond
by swinging in the opposite direction in an effort to rebalance itself. If a
body is operating efficiently, it will regain equilibrium quickly and come
to rest at the center point.

But what if the body is in a state of disease? This can be viewed as a
pendulum that is stuck off center (see figure). The body will feel out of
whack, and things won't be functioning and reacting normally. For
example, a person might manifest a severely allergic response to a benign
substance, with the pendulum swinging wildly out of proportion to the

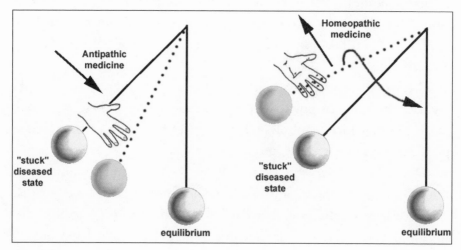

Pendulum Model

stimulus. Or, instead of dealing with the natural ups and downs of life in a balanced way, the psyche may become stuck in a distorted stance toward life, causing it to react in inappropriate ways.

One way to understand the difference between allopathy and homeopathy is to look at how they deal with the "stuck pendulum." The antipathic approach (the approach largely used by allopaths) is to forcibly push the pendulum back toward the center position. For example, antidepressants are used to force the brain out of its depressive state. In contrast, the homeopathic approach is to give the pendulum a very slight nudge in the opposite (diseased) direction. By providing the vital force with an energetic stimulus that is similar to the diseased state, a homeopathic remedy enables the pendulum to become "unstuck" and to respond by swinging back toward equilibrium.

The pendulum model may also explain why homeopathic remedies are able to cure rather than merely palliate. A remedy enables the pendulum to move in the curative direction *on its own.* While it is the remedy that enables the pendulum to become unstuck, it is the body and the vital force that actually move the pendulum back toward equilibrium. In contrast, antipathic medicines artificially force the pendulum toward the center position. When the external antipathic agent is removed, the pendulum eventually creeps back toward its accustomed diseased state; in some cases, it may even react and become stuck even further away from equilibrium.

Here's a little experiment that you can perform to test the action-counteraction model for yourself. It turns out that the homeopathic approach to dealing with burns is to apply *heat* rather than cold to the site of a burn. How could this possibly work? It works because the body naturally responds to the application of heat by later cooling itself — action/counteraction. Check it out for yourself. Take two buckets of water, one very cold, the other hot, but not hot enough to burn you. Put your hand in the cold bucket for 15 seconds and then take it out. What happens? Your hand will start to feel very hot. Now put your other hand in the hot bucket for 15 seconds. Afterward, you will find that your hand will start to feel very cold.

Now, test it out in practice. The next time you get a minor burn in the kitchen, don't use cold water. Cold water may make the burn feel better while it's under the water, but later on the burn will become even hotter and hurt even more. Instead, put your burn under very warm water — as warm as you can tolerate for 10 or 15 seconds. Now see what happens. I have been using this response to kitchen burns for a few years now, and I have not once developed a blister. In fact, within minutes, I usually do not have any sign of a burn at all. I have also heard that workers who routinely operate near severe heat use the homeopathic strategy as well. For example, glass blowers and cooks know that the appropriate response to a burn is to hold the burn near the fire in order to heat it. After this brief application of heat, the body will naturally overcool the burned area and heal it faster. One chef wrote:

> "I have spent eight years as a chef, burning myself at least once a night...When you are cooking in a restaurant there is no time to stop and nurse your burn, you must continue to keep your hands over the heat. I have found that this process of *gently* heating the burn actually takes the pain away and heals the burn more quickly. Ice brings immediate relief, but seems to prolong the pain and the healing process... The key here is not to continue to burn yourself but to heat the area gently." [SL1]

2. Energetic Strengthening Through Resonance

I have already discussed George Vithoulkas's conception of the vital force as an energetic field resonating at a particular frequency. One way of looking at a homeopathic remedy is as a substance that resonates at the same frequency as the patient, and as a result, strengthens or amplifies their vital force, enabling it to heal once again. In essence, the remedy boosts the vital force, and consequently, the immune system as well. Vithoulkas writes,

> "To affect directly the dynamic plane, we must find a substance similar enough to the resultant frequency of the dynamic plane to produce resonance... If a substance is capable of producing a similar symptom picture in a healthy organism, then the likelihood of its vibration rate being very close to the resultant frequency of the diseased organism is

good, and therefore a powerful strengthening of the defense mechanism can occur — through the principle of resonance." [Vithoulkas, p. 91]

(Copyright © 1980 by George Vithoulkas. Used by permission of Grove/Atlantic, Inc.)

The resonance between a remedy and a patient's vital force can be likened to two violin strings vibrating at the same frequency that resonate and amplify one another. The remedy (violin string) that will resonate the best with a diseased patient (other violin string) is the one that can produce the same symptoms being experienced by that patient — i.e., the one that is homeopathic to the patient's state. Another way of looking at this is that people and remedies with the same vibration tend to create the same symptoms.

This conception of the homeopathic principle is also probably what underlies the success of psychological support groups. The people who participate in such groups are experiencing similar problems and therefore resonate together to create healing. This "psychological homeopathy" is quite familiar to homeopaths and was even discussed by Hahnemann in the *Organon*, long before the advent of modern-day psychology.

3. Distracting or Fooling the Vital Force: Disease Replacement
Another way of looking at the action of a remedy is as a kind of distraction or ruse that fools the vital force. If susceptibility can be viewed as a gap or hole that is filled by disease, one way of curing that susceptibility is to fill the gap with something else — something very similar to the disease: a homeopathic remedy. When the gap in the vital force is filled by the remedy rather than by the disease, its needs are met and it loses its susceptibility. But because the remedy "disease" is merely artificial, functioning as a disease facade, it soon fades away of its own accord. And now that the person's need for the disease has been fulfilled, his or her vital force also loses its susceptibility. Note the similarity of this model to Bellavite and Signorini's notion of the remedy serving as an alternate attractor that guides the body away from a disease attractor.

How exactly is the disease energy displaced from the hole of susceptibility? One way to imagine this is to think about how magnets work. The energy of the remedy might repel and dislodge the energy of the disease, much as the north poles of two magnets repel each other. This happens because the energies of the remedy and the disease are similar. Although Hahnemann didn't place much importance on the need for a model of remedy action, this "disease replacement" model was one of his favorites. He wrote:

> "This natural law of cure [the Law of Similars] has authenticated itself to the world in all pure experiments and all genuine experiences; therefore it exists as fact. Scientific explanations for *how it takes place* do not matter very much and I do not attach much importance to attempts made to explain it. The following view, however, is verifiably the most probable since it is based on nothing but empirical premises:
>
> 1. Any disease (which is not strictly a surgical case) consists solely of a specific dynamic disease mistunement of our life force... in our feelings and functions.
>
> 2. The life principle, which has been dynamically mistuned by the natural disease, is *seized*, during homeopathic cure, by the similar yet somewhat stronger artificial disease-affection which results from the application of the medicinal potence [remedy], selected exactly according to symptom similarity.
>
> 3. The feeling of the natural (weaker) dynamic disease-affection [the original natural disease] is extinguished and disappears for the life principle and, from then on, no longer exists for the life principle...
>
> 4. The artificial disease-affection [from the remedy] soon plays itself out, leaving the patient free and recuperated. The dynamis, thus freed, can now continue life again, in health." [Hahnemann, Aphorisms 28 and 29]

Jungian psychiatrist Edward Whitmont, MD, believed that various phenomena in psychiatric medicine give support to the disease replacement model as well. For example, certain mental conditions are known to correspond and fluidly interchange with specific physical ailments. Whitmont believed that symptoms migrate between physical and psychological realms because they mirror one another. In his book, *Psyche and Substance,* he links this phenomenon to the action of homeopathic remedies. Just as a mental condition can replace a physical one, or vice versa, Whitmont viewed the homeopathic remedy as a kind of temporary replacement for a disease state. But by being able to replace it, a remedy can also ultimately remove disease completely. He wrote:

> "...with mental and physical symptoms synchronistically, not causally, related, one may substitute for another and appear to be able to cancel it. Thus we get a first glimpse of an understanding how illness and 'similar' drug energy, as synchronistic entities of the same 'field' sharing a functional likeness, may perhaps substitute for another and thereby functionally cancel each other." [Whitmont, p. 86]

As Hahnemann pointed out, the disease replacement model of remedy action is also backed up by clinical experience. For example, it explains why a remedy whose effects are most similar to the disease state works best (it is the best counterfeit disease), and why a weakly matching remedy only palliates for a while and may even create auxiliary symptoms (the vital force has not really lost its susceptibility, and the parts of the remedy that don't "fit" just spill over). This model may also explain why slowly increasing the potency of a remedy works so well. A gradual increase in potency enables the vital force to become more and more completely fooled, the natural disease to be more surely displaced, and the susceptibility to be filled more completely.

Another way that I like to think about this model of remedy action is as a kind of gradual coaxing or leading of the vital force away from an accustomed disease posture. Imagine that the diseased vital force is a creature that is hiding in a place that it is afraid to leave. If the creature is provided a different place to go to, a place that seems similar to its favorite spot, it might be lured out. Very slowly, as the true nature of its new location comes into greater focus, the creature will realize that it has left its hiding place. But by now, it will also have been cured of its fixation. This experience, this feeling of being led out of the "stuck place" and suddenly becoming clear and cognizant of having been trapped there, is something that many cured homeopathic patients report.

4. Remedy as Information

As I have already described, the action of remedies can be viewed in terms of information and complexity theory [Bellavite]. In particular, a remedy can be seen as providing just the right piece of information to create the appropriate effects in the complex systems of the body. One can also view the information provided by a remedy in symbolic terms. If disease is the vital force in a state of delusion or erroneous belief, a remedy is the truth-giver that finally provides the vital force with correct information so that it can do its job once again.

Homeopaths have used a variety of analogies and metaphors for an informational view of remedy action. Jeremy Sherr, an Israeli-British homeopath, tells it like this. Being in a state of disease is like driving down the right highway in the wrong direction. The driver knows that he is on the right road, but he never reaches his destination. Perhaps he is looking in the rearview mirror rather than the front windshield — his perception is off. The remedy is a voice that tells the driver: "Hey, you're going in the wrong direction!" When the driver first hears this, he might get very upset (experience an aggravation of symptoms). But if the car has enough gas (the body has a strong enough vital force), the driver can turn around and go in the right direction. While doing so, he will pass all the places he has already been (experience a reversal of symptoms).

Another metaphor likens the vital force to an army. The army is trying to do the best job it can. But without proper intelligence, it may simply be operating ineffectively. The remedy is like an informant that tells the army what's really going on. It presents an accurate view of the disease (the enemy) to the vital force: "Here is what is happening. *This* is your foe." Supplied with this correct information, the army can now do its job.

Hahnemann also used the army analogy, and coupled it with the notion of a remedy as a strengthening agent. He wrote:

> "If we physicians are able to present and oppose to this instinctive vital force its morbific enemy, as it were magnified through the action of homeopathic medicines — if in this way the image of the morbific foe

be magnified to the apprehension of the vital principle..., we gradually cause and compel this instinctive vital force to increase its energies
by degrees, and to increase them more and more, and at last to such a
degree that it becomes far more powerful than the original disease. The
consequence of this is that the vital force again becomes sovereign in
its domain." [HahnemannCD, p. xviii]

One final analogy is of a more spiritual nature. Disease is viewed as
a form of disconnect from God, the life source. The remedy is the
required link — a piece of information that enables the vital force to
reconnect once again with the divine. One patient summarized her six-
month experience of homeopathic healing much like this:

> "I have my spirit back — my inner light. Before, when I was hopeless,
> I could not connect with it... I believe whatever this remedy did, I felt
> alone and abandoned by God and the remedy connected me up to the
> light... I think that the wound that happens to most people is separa-
> tion from the spirit. It's the disconnect — the human condition from
> the spirit. Homeopathy is a simple way, there is no need for 20 years
> of psychotherapy. It goes straight through things. Since I took the rem-
> edy I feel bigger inside... There is an expansiveness to the remedy. That
> remedy must have some amazing vibration. It's astounding! Nothing
> will stop homeopathy now — if people have experiences like mine
> they'll shout it from the rooftops." [Melnychuk, pp. 123–124]

PUTTING IT ALL TOGETHER

How to put all of these ideas together? Homeopathic models and scientific experiments provide us with clues, but they are probably only partial
views of the whole truth. The explanation for how homeopathy truly
works is surely something that incorporates all of these ideas and more.
Here is my own attempt at synthesizing many of these concepts together.

Disease comes upon us when our vital force becomes stuck in a state
that is no longer an appropriate adaptation to the physical and emotional requirements of life. The reason for this is usually some emotional or
physical event, or perhaps many such events. Somehow, the vital force was

susceptible to these events and couldn't adapt. As a result, it is now struggling, blocked, or warped in some way. Over time, this perturbed energetic state causes perceptible emotional, mental, and physical symptoms.

The remedy, by holding a similar vibration to our own diseased state, is able to resonate with us and provide exactly the right piece of information to the vital force so that it starts moving properly again. Our vital force is everywhere in and around our body, and our body is largely water. If this information touches the body and its vital force, it will quickly permeate them.

Once the remedy information has been transmitted, a process of normalization of the vital force begins. This normalization may occur in slow gradual steps and require lots of little nudges and reminders via contact with the resonant remedy, or it may happen very quickly — almost instantaneously. Normalization of the vital force enables it to finally respond as it should — with counteraction to the disease disturbance. And with this counteraction comes the concomitant healing on the mental, emotional, and physical planes.

Of course, since healing with homeopathy is actually the work of our own vital force, it may take time for that force to direct the physical body and mind back toward health. It might even take months or years. But if the vital force has the energy — if it is strong enough to enable the body and mind to become sound once more — healing will take place. And because this healing is actually *self-healing,* it will feel quite different from allopathic treatment that is forced. After all, being shoved into a new state of being feels quite different than entering into it naturally.

Ideally, the experience of homeopathic healing is like the one described by the patient who felt reconnected with her spirit — a feeling of discovering one's true nature again, great relief, and happiness. The next chapter will discuss this healing process in more detail — what the experience of homeopathy is all about.

CHAPTER 8

*

THE EXPERIENCE OF
HOMEOPATHY

"The diagnosis of disease by modern methods [allopathy] is based largely upon physical signs, tests and reactions, involving the use of many
instruments of precision, in which the patient takes no active part, and
of which he has no knowledge. The selection of the homoeopathic remedy, on the other hand, is based very largely and sometimes almost
entirely upon the phenomena... of subjective, conscious experience, per-
ceived only by the patient and stated by him to the examiner."

— Stuart Close, MD, *The Genius of Homeopathy*, 1924 [Close]

MOST PEOPLE GET THEIR FIRST TASTE OF HOMEOPATHY BY
trying an over-the-counter remedy for some minor ailment.
Another common entryway is first aid — for instance, using Arnica for
bumps and bruises, or *Calendula* (made from marigold) as a topical oint-
ment. Many then take the next step and try their hand at self-treatment,
using one of the many excellent homeopathic self-help books available
— for example, Miranda Castro's *Complete Homeopathy Handbook* [Castro].
This can be a great low-cost way to meet many family health needs — if
used judiciously.

The best way to pursue homeopathic treatment, however, is under
the care of an experienced, trained homeopath. While some ailments may
seem minor — for example, allergies or sinus problems — they can also
be signs of a deeper problem that could be cured homeopathically, not
just palliated. To find this kind of deeper cure, patients must see a home-

opath. So where to begin? And what to expect? This chapter will guide you as you pursue the experience of homeopathy — from finding a homeopath and preparing for your first appointment, to knowing what to expect as you travel the path toward cure.

SELECTING A HOMEOPATH

Finding a good homeopath may take a little work. First, try word of mouth. You may be acquainted with a local chiropractor, osteopath, or acupuncturist. Such practitioners are often aware of homeopaths local to their area. Other places to inquire are health food stores and the phone book (look under "Homeopath" or "Holistic Practitioners"). The Internet is also a good resource. If you are seeking a classical homeopath in the United States or Canada, check *www.homeopathicdirectory.com* for a listing of certified practitioners. Another excellent referral list is located at *www.homeopathy-cures.com*. For those readers living elsewhere in the world, start by visiting a site that is a good starting point for all things homeopathic: *www.homeopathyhome.com*. If you click on Directory, you will be led to country-specific practitioner lists.

The national homeopathic organizations are also good places to look for information. For example, the National Center for Homeopathy (NCH) publishes a membership list that highlights members who are practitioners. Because this listing is self-referred, however, these practitioners may or may not have been assessed for competency. Check practitioner credentials to see if they are certified in homeopathy. The NCH also has many affiliated study groups. Contacting a study group local to your area is another great way to find a practitioner. The NCH can be contacted at:

National Center for Homeopathy
801 North Fairfax Street, Suite 306
Alexandria, Virginia 22314
877-624-0613 (toll free)
info@homeopathic.org
www.homeopathic.org

Another organization is the North American Society of Homeopaths (NASH), a professional society representing homeopaths in the United States and Canada whose members hold the title RSHom (NA). Most NASH members are professional homeopaths — i.e., practitioners who have completed comprehensive homeopathic training programs and have met certification standards, but do not hold medical licensure. (There are no states that offer licensure for homeopathy; licensed practitioners must hold a license in some other medical profession.) NASH has recently opened up its membership to include licensed practitioners as well, as long as they have been certified by the Council for Homeopathic Certification (CHC). This council awards the CCH credential. NASH and the CHC can be reached at the addresses below.

North American Society of Homeopaths
1122 East Pike Street #1122
Seattle, Washington 98122
206-720-7000
nashinfo@aol.com
www.homeopathy.org

Council for Homeopathic Certification
PMB 187
17051 SE 272nd Street, Suite #43
Covington, Washington 98042
866-242-3399 (toll free)
chcinfo@homeopathicdirectory.com
www.homeopathicdirectory.com

As mentioned in Chapter 1, some licensed doctors, osteopaths, and naturopaths have also begun to specialize in homeopathy. For example, a DHt certification (Diplomate in Homeotherapeutics) is available to MDs and DOs and is awarded by the American Board of Homeotherapeutics. You can find more information about this organization by contacting the National Center for Homeopathy or by checking the web site: *www.homeopathyusa.org/specialtyboard*. The small group of naturopaths who specialize in homeopathy (currently, around 50 naturopaths) are members of the Homeopathic Academy of Naturopathic Physicians (HANP) and hold the DHANP certification. The HANP can be reached at:

Homeopathic Academy for Naturopathic Physicians
1412 W. Washington Street
Boise, Idaho 83702
208-336-3390
info@hanp.net
www.hanp.net

Once you have selected a potential homeopath, it is a good idea to interview them on the telephone. This will enable you to find out if their personal philosophy and style of homeopathic practice matches your expectations. You might ask if they use single remedies or polypharmacy, how long their initial interview takes (most classical homeopaths will conduct an interview that takes at least one hour, sometimes two hours), and whether they handle acute as well as chronic care. Beware of practitioners who use devices to select a remedy or to "measure" your energy field. These are usually not classically trained homeopaths, even if they dispense remedies.

Another way to evaluate a potential homeopath is to ask for patient references. This can be helpful in determining what a practitioner is like as a person and how accessible they are. Remember: it is important to find a practitioner that you can feel comfortable with. A homeopath will not be able to help you unless you are able to fully reveal your psychological and physical case history to them.

PREPARING FOR YOUR FIRST VISIT

I opened this chapter with a quote from *The Genius of Homoeopathy*, a homeopathic philosophy text written by turn-of-the-20th-century homeopath Stuart Close, MD. As Close points out, most of the data that homeopaths use in making remedy choices are provided by their patients. Thus, to receive good homeopathic care, you must be an active and communicative participant in the healing process. Laboratory tests and physical measuring devices, while perhaps useful in assessing the severity of an illness, are generally unhelpful in homeopathic prescribing. Indeed, unlicensed practitioners are not even allowed to order such tests.

The primary mode of interaction between you and your homeopath will therefore be verbal; you will sit and talk about your physical and emotional symptoms for one or two hours. Indeed, this interview may seem much more like a visit to a psychologist than to a physician. Most homeopaths charge for their services in much the same way as psychologists do as well — by the hour, and usually at about the same rate. However, it is not unusual for a homeopath to charge a slightly higher rate for the first interview. This is because initial remedy selection requires additional study and analysis, some of which may take place after your appointment. Subsequent follow-up visits are generally shorter in length and are charged at a lower rate.

Since the quality of your homeopathic care will be largely dependent on the information you provide, it is a good idea to prepare for your first visit. Some homeopaths facilitate this process by having clients fill out a questionnaire in advance. A typical questionnaire covers details like diet and food preferences, medications or supplements being taken, and medical history. In addition to filling out this questionnaire, I advise that you jot down observations that you can make about yourself. One useful exercise is to carry around a sheet of paper with you for a day or two before your appointment and record any odd habits or symptoms that you may have become accustomed to and therefore might not otherwise notice or remember. For example, do you have congestion when you wake up in the morning or at night in bed? Do you have a particular pattern of sweating, perhaps on your head or chest? Do you have a tendency to become itchy at certain times of the day? Do you have fears in certain situations — for instance, a fear of heights, dogs, water, or of being alone? What have your dreams been like lately?

For every symptom, try to determine if it is made worse or better by something. Such factors are called symptom *modalities*. For example, you might find that you tend to be itchy just after you remove your clothes at night, that you cough whenever you inhale cold air, or that your asthma improves in the summer. Other kinds of modalities that may ameliorate or aggravate your symptoms are the following:

- *Certain times of day or seasons of the year.*
- *Weather such as rain, fog, storms, dry heat, wind, etc.*
- *Emotional or social situations.*
- *Movements or positions of the body, such as sitting, lying, bending, or walking.*
- *Certain kinds of clothing.*
- *Eating certain foods.*
- *Pressure, heat, or cold.*
- *Reactions to certain locales, such as stuffy rooms, the mountains, or the seaside.*

It is also important to try to determine the exact nature of each symptom — how it evolved over time, what its sensation is like, where it occurs, whether or not it extends to other parts of your body, and if it is consistently accompanied by other symptoms. For example, is your headache pulsating, stabbing, or bursting? Is it in the back of your head, on top of your head, or over an eye? Is it accompanied by thirst or sensitivity to light or noise? Is it worse after eating, or at particular times of the day? Have you found that most of your symptoms occur on one side of your body? Are most of your symptoms aggravated or ameliorated by the same thing? Were your symptoms triggered by a particular physical or emotional event? Of course, your homeopath will also ask questions during your appointment to help you fill out these symptom details.

Here is an additional checklist of things to help you prepare for an appointment. Try not to get bogged down in too much detail. Only note a symptom if it is pronounced and persistent, and especially, if it is unusual. And don't forget to record symptom modalities — i.e., the things that make a symptom worse or better.

- *Go over your body from head to toe* and notice any unusual sensations you may be experiencing. Include headaches or any other aches and pains.

- *Problems with the senses* (vision, hearing, smell, taste, touch, and vertigo).

- *Digestive, bowel, and urinary symptoms.* How is your appetite? Do you tend to be thirsty or thirstless? Are you experiencing indigestion, or bowel problems such as constipation or diarrhea? Is your urinary function unusual? Is it difficult to pass urine or feces in particular situations? Is your stool or urine unusual in heat, color, or form? Do you have hemorrhoids? Is it difficult to swallow liquids or solids? Are you experiencing excessive belching, flatulence, or nausea?

- *Respiratory symptoms.* Are you experiencing difficulties with breathing, coughing, or asthma? Are you bringing up unusual amounts of phlegm?

- *Circulatory symptoms.* Do you have chest pains or other heart problems? Are your extremities excessively cold or hot? Do you tend to be hot or cold in general?

- *Neurological symptoms.* Are you experiencing tremors, twitching, convulsions, numbness, or paralysis of any kind?

- *Sexual function.* Women should review their past menstrual history, current menstrual pattern, any problems experienced during childbirth, and their use of contraception or hormonal supplements. Both men and women should think about problems with sexual desire (both excessive or diminished), and whether they are experiencing discharges of any kind. Also important to review are sexually transmitted diseases you currently have or have experienced in the past.

- *Skin eruptions, ulcerations, itching, and sweating patterns.*

- *Food desires and aversions.* These should be genuine and marked preferences and aversions — i.e., what you truly like or hate to eat, not what you think you should eat.

- *Birth details.* For young children, note anything unusual experienced during conception, gestation, or childbirth. Include physical and emotional events that impacted the child's parents during this period.

- *Sleep and dreams.* What position do you sleep in? Do you like to sleep with the windows open or closed, or with the covers on or off particular parts of your body? Do you have any problems with sleeping? What is your typical pattern of waking and falling asleep? Do you talk or walk in your sleep? Do you snore or sweat? What makes your sleep problems worse or better? What dreams have you been having? Are there any recurrent dreams?

- *Problems with depression, oversensitivity, learning disabilities, or any other emotional, behavioral, or cognitive disturbance.*

Of course, in addition to all of these symptoms, a homeopath is interested in what you are like as a person. What is your life story? What are your habits, fears, aspirations, and hobbies, and what problems are you having at work or in your relationships? What kind of person are you? How do others perceive you? Do you tend to be suspicious, jealous, bossy, friendly, submissive, irritable, easily hurt, restless, or lethargic? You may find that the bulk of your first interview is filled with relating this kind of information. That's why it helps to jot down your physical symptoms and modalities in advance — so that they can be covered more quickly, and so that you don't forget to relate important physical information once you have started talking about your life as a whole. You can also contact your homeopath after your interview if you forgot to mention key details. If a homeopath feels they need more information from you, they may contact you after your appointment as well.

THE INTERVIEW

It's the day of your first interview with your homeopath. What can you expect? Most homeopaths practice in small office settings. Like psychologists, they take notes as you speak. Since most practitioners utilize computers for performing case analysis, they may type their interview notes directly into a computer, as you speak. This may be a bit disconcerting at first, but rest assured, they are listening. Among other things, homeopaths are trained to take very seriously the way you express yourself. They may even type in or write down many of the things you say verbatim. Some homeopaths may ask for permission to record your interview on audio- or videotape as well.

Of course, a major difference between a psychotherapeutic visit and a homeopathic visit is the underlying goal of the practitioner. A homeopath is trying to learn enough about you in order to select a good remedy. It is not their goal to cure you through conversation. As a result, the homeopathic interview may seem somewhat one-sided. You will relate all you need to say, and the homeopath will speak relatively little, except to inquire about more information. Try to be as cooperative and as forthcoming as you can, knowing that the more truthful and open you are, the better the chance that your health problems will be solved.

The process of case analysis and remedy selection can begin once your homeopath feels they have understood the major elements of your case. Since this may happen in the middle of your interview, don't be disturbed if they suddenly start navigating around a computer program. Just keep talking — the details you provide will continue to aid in their analysis. Most homeopaths who perform case analysis during the interview will also try to recommend a remedy by the end of the appointment. Other homeopaths prefer to conduct their analysis after the interview and will recommend a remedy a few days later. Additional time for case analysis may also be required for complex cases.

CASE ANALYSIS TOOLS

So what exactly is the homeopath doing as they analyze a case? Chapter 5 discussed several aspects of this process. I will now review that discussion and provide some additional detail.

After collecting a patient's symptoms, a homeopath uses two kinds of resources to choose a remedy for a patient, both of which are now available in computerized form. Indeed, the computer has revolutionized the modern practice of homeopathy, making it incredibly more efficient and flexible than was possible in the past. The primary homeopathic resource is the *materia medica* — a reference that contains a compendium of information about each remedy. Each remedy description includes hundreds of symptoms of body, mind, and emotions that have been gathered during proving trials or have been cured clinically with that remedy. Over the past two hundred years, homeopaths have compiled scores of materia medica in book form. Today, all of these books, as well as information about new provings, are available digitally. Using powerful search engines and databases, quick and flexible access to a wealth of information is right at a homeopath's fingertips.

The second kind of homeopathic resource is a reverse index to the materia medica called a *repertory*. A repertory contains a listing of symptoms, organized in a methodical way. Associated with each symptom is a list of remedies that include that symptom. These are the remedies that have caused that symptom in a proving, or have consistently cured that symptom in practice. Each "symptom/remedy–list" pair is called a *rubric*.

For example, one of the classic repertories was compiled by James T. Kent, MD, an American homeopath of the late 1800s and early 1900s [KentRep]. It is organized into chapters, each pertaining to different parts, functions, and systems of the body. These include chapters on the Mind (mental and emotional symptoms), Vertigo, Head, Vision (symptoms of vision), Eyes (symptoms of the eyes themselves), Hearing, Ears, Nose, Mouth, Throat, Chest, Stomach, Abdomen, Back, Rectum, Urinary Tract, Genitals (including menstrual function and childbirth), Respiratory System, Extremities, Sleep, and Skin. Each of these chapters contains a list of rubrics, each of which may be subdivided into more detailed rubrics.

For instance, in the Stomach chapter of Kent's repertory, we have a variety of heartburn rubrics, at increasing degrees of specificity — i.e., each is modified by more and more specific circumstances in which heartburn occurs. For example, consider the following rubrics:

STOMACH, Heartburn   <remedy list A>

evening   <remedy list B>

smoking, after   <remedy list C>

All of the remedies in list *A* are associated with the general symptom of heartburn. Remedies in list *B* are those in which heartburn occurs in the evening. Finally, remedies in list *C* are those in which heartburn occurs in the evening after smoking. As one might expect, the more unique and odd a symptom is, the fewer the remedies that will be associated with it. In the rubric example above, remedy list *A* has 118 remedies in it, remedy list *B* has 11, and remedy list *C* has only 1 remedy (*Lachesis,* made from the poison of the bushmaster snake).

The remedies within each rubric are also graded or ranked according to the intensity of the association between the remedy and the symptom. Each grade is identified either by a number (usually 1–4) or by typeface. For example, a boldface or capitalized remedy indicates that it has a high grade. This rating system enables a homeopath to evaluate remedy choices in a more detailed way. For instance, if a symptom is very strong in a patient's case, it is also desirable that a candidate remedy manifest that symptom very strongly as well.

REPERTORIZATION AND REMEDY SELECTION

Armed with good case information, a materia medica, and a repertory, a homeopath begins case analysis by selecting the most essential symptoms of the case. This also happens to be the hardest part of case analysis and requires the most experience. An accomplished homeopath will usually be able to pick four or five key symptoms to analyze — those symptoms that will most likely lead to a good remedy choice. A less experienced homeopath may grapple with dozens of symptoms and find it hard to weed out the most important ones.

Once a set of symptoms has been selected, each must be translated into a rubric or set of rubrics. Then, computerized repertory programs can be used to automatically find the remedies that appear in all of the rubrics, or at least in most of them. The result is a smaller set of remedies that the homeopath must now consider in greater detail. He or she will study each of these remedies in the materia medica, and, ideally, one remedy will emerge as the best choice.

One can imagine how tedious this process must have been in the days before computers. Special "repertory sheets" were used to intersect large sets of remedies manually; a process that takes seconds today would take hours a hundred years ago. Computers have also made today's case analysis much more flexible and powerful than was possible before. For example, computer programs enable a homeopath to focus on specific remedy groups (specific types of animals, plants, or minerals); to assign stronger or weaker weights to specific symptoms; and to search directly for symptom keywords in the materia medica and proving records.

If your homeopath conducts their analysis during your appointment, they will probably ask you some additional questions to confirm their remedy choice. For example, don't be surprised if, at the end of your interview, your homeopath asks you something odd like, "Do you by any chance get diarrhea from eating potatoes?" If you do indeed avoid potatoes for just this reason, you may think that he or she is nothing short of psychic! But the truth is, it only means that they have found an excellent remedy choice for you — one that also happens to include your sensitivity to potatoes.

If your homeopath makes a remedy selection for you by the end of your appointment, they will also explain how to acquire and take the remedy. Some practitioners stock their own remedies and provide them to clients at very low cost; others have clients order remedies from a homeopathic pharmacy. But do not be disappointed if your homeopath says that they need a few extra days to study your case before they can make a remedy recommendation. The additional time they take will help to ensure that the chosen remedy will be beneficial for you.

TAKING YOUR REMEDY

Chapter 6 discussed the various methods of remedy administration in detail. Your homeopath will probably recommend either a *dry dose* (tiny white pills) or a *liquid dose*, in which pills are dissolved in a mixture of water and a small amount of alcohol (as a preservative). The dosing method chosen for you will depend on your homeopath's personal dosing preferences, the details of your case, other treatments that you are taking, and the potency selected for you. The possibilities are actually quite broad. Your homeopath may instruct you to take a single dry dose (i.e., one tiny pill) and nothing more. Or, you might be told to take two or three pills several times a day over a period of days. Liquid dosing may be administered daily, weekly, or as symptoms warrant.

Whatever type of dosing is recommended for you, follow your homeopath's instructions precisely. If you are uncertain about these instructions, call your homeopath on the phone. When you actually take a dose, avoid eating or drinking anything for a period of time (at least 10–15 minutes) before or afterward. This enables the energy of the remedy to permeate your system with the least amount of interference. For dry doses, simply let the pills melt in your mouth. Since they are made of sugar impregnated with the remedy, they will even taste nice. You will have no problem getting children to take them. It is also best if pills are handled only by the person who is taking them.

Liquid dosing requires a bit more care. You will probably be instructed to perform a certain number of succussions (vigorous shakes) to the remedy bottle before each dose. After succussion, take the prescribed amount from the bottle (usually a teaspoon or a drop from a dropper bottle) and put it into yet another glass of water (usually ¼ to ½ cup of water) and stir. Finally, administer the prescribed dose (usually a teaspoon) from this glass. The frequency of doses, the number of succussions used, and the physical amount administered each time will vary depending on your response to the remedy. Ask your homeopath for written instructions.

Finally, when it comes to dosing, try to remember that *more is not better* in homeopathy. In fact, *less is better.* I have heard of patients who, instead of taking a single teaspoon from a bottle, drank the whole bottle and then suffered an unnecessary aggravation. It is also not uncommon to hear about people who, upon amelioration of their symptoms after a single dose, keep taking more. If you can remember only one piece of advice, remember this:

> *If your symptoms are improving, do nothing. Do not take another dose unless your symptoms are getting worse again. When in doubt, do nothing, and call your homeopath.*

Most of us who are accustomed to allopathic treatment believe that we need to keep taking drugs in order to get the desired effect. This may be appropriate with allopathic drugs, since they force the body into a state that is unnatural to it and therefore must be maintained. In contrast, homeopathic remedies coax the body to repair itself. Once this process has been set into motion, it should be left to proceed on its own. Only in those cases where a disease does not yield easily or where it quickly relapses should a remedy (especially a dry dose) be repeated. If your body seems to be healing, don't rock the boat.

ANTIDOTING

Most homeopaths provide patients with a list of substances and practices to avoid while they are undergoing homeopathic treatment. The reason for this is the potential problem of *antidoting* — i.e., the possibility that some other substance or activity will nullify or lessen the effects of a remedy.

In general, antidotal factors are things that tend to affect the body and vital force in strong ways. The most common antidotes are coffee, strong-smelling perfumes or mints, camphor, other drugs and supplements (recreational or medicinal), dental visits, and the use of hormone replacement or birth control pills. Obviously, you will not be able to avoid all of these things all of the time, so discuss the issue of antidoting with your homeopath if you have concerns or questions. Whether or not something will actually antidote your treatment will depend on your individual characteristics. The basic determinant is how susceptible you are to the potential antidote. For example, if you tend to be severely affected by dental appointments and suffer physical or emotional aftereffects, you will also be more likely antidoted by a dental visit. If dental visits are usually no problem, it is unlikely that they will antidote your treatment.

Of course, most people are not easily antidoted at all. For example, drinking a cup of coffee has never antidoted my own homeopathic treatment (although my craving for coffee diminished and I have stopped drinking it). However, some people are very susceptible to coffee, and may even be antidoted by simply walking into a coffee shop and smelling the strong coffee aromas. For this reason, most homeopaths will request all of their patients to avoid the most common antidotal factors, especially coffee and camphor, whenever possible.

But why is there potential for antidoting at all? Remember that homeopathy is a subtle energy medicine that enables your vital force to shift away from a faulty posture. This shift is enabled by the small energetic nudge supplied by the remedy, and once it has taken place, it is maintained by the strength of your vital force. If you simultaneously bombard yourself with strong influences that sap your energy and vitality, you will also sap away the beneficial changes that a remedy has set in motion.

Think of it this way. Suppose that you would like to quit smoking or drinking. An ideal way to do this would be to take a holiday and get away from life's stresses. A relaxed and wholesome atmosphere gives the body a chance to rest and enhances its ability to take on new habits and repair itself. The longer you can maintain this new lifestyle, the more likely you'll be able to keep away from cigarettes or alcohol.

But what's the chance that you will be able to quit smoking or drinking if you keep bombarding yourself with stresses? Very small. The same goes for your vital force. To create the optimum chance for positive remedy effects, try to keep your life as clean and as stress-free as possible. Obviously, this will also benefit your health. But rest assured, homeopathy *can* work even when your life can't be made stress-free. In fact, it is common wisdom among homeopaths that the closer a remedy is to the patient's simillimum, the less likely that anything will be able to antidote it.

REMEDY RESPONSE

Once you've started taking a remedy, what should you expect?

An ideal response to a homeopathic remedy should go something like this. First, you will feel a general improvement in your sense of well-being. Perhaps your sleep improves, your mental state and emotional outlook brightens, your vitality goes up, your digestion improves and your bowels move more regularly, or your menstrual cycle becomes more regular. A good remedy response may even affect seemingly unrelated aspects of your life. For example, you may suddenly become more lucky in life. You meet the man or woman of your dreams, you get a raise at work, or your schoolwork improves. These things happen because, in the course of true healing, your whole energetic field will be changed for the better. This change will enable the people around you to respond better to you as well.

Although you may initially feel better in general, a good remedy response may also involve a short period of aggravation of your chronic complaint — perhaps a few days, or even a couple of weeks. During this period you may also experience a brief "cleansing" reaction — usually a discharge of some kind. It might be diarrhea, nasal discharge, or the eruption of a skin rash. Try not to suppress these reactions with allopathic medicines.

Finally, after a brief period of aggravation (which may or may not occur), your chronic complaint will also begin to improve, perhaps slowly and gradually, but nevertheless, in a continuous path of improvement.

You may find that a stressful day sets you back a bit, but afterward, you resume your path toward recovery. If you have a complex health history, you may find that some old complaints from the past return, especially if they were suppressed by allopathic treatment. Try not to suppress these symptoms again. They might disappear on their own after a few days, or they may yield to further homeopathic treatment. Call your homeopath if you have any questions.

Please note that the remedy reactions I have just described are characteristic of treatment for *chronic* complaints. In acute cases such as viral or bacterial infections, this process is compressed. First of all, aggravations do not usually occur. Instead, a curative response is usually heralded by the person falling asleep, or falling asleep after first vomiting. Recovery should then proceed quickly — often within hours. If it does not, further treatment with additional doses or other remedies may be warranted.

What about not-so-ideal reactions?

If you experience a strong aggravation of your chronic complaint, but otherwise do not develop any completely new symptoms, the potency of the remedy you took was probably incorrect or the amount of remedy you took was too large. In this situation, your homeopath may decide to prescribe another potency of the same remedy to alleviate your reaction (in some cases a lower potency, in other cases a higher potency). Most likely, however, your homeopath will ask you to simply not take any more doses and to stick with the aggravation a bit longer to see if it passes on its own. Rest assured that an aggravation of this kind is a sign that the remedy has touched your vital force and that you will experience relief after a few days.

If you experience a general decline in health, or if all new and severe symptoms appear and persist, it is a sign that an incorrect remedy has been given and in too large a dose. Indeed, even if your chronic complaint has improved, a general worsening in health means that the complaint has been suppressed rather than cured. If you are taking regular doses of your remedy, discontinue it and call your homeopath. After discontinuing the remedy, these new and troublesome symptoms should subside. If they do not, your homeopath may decide to prescribe a new remedy, or may ask you to antidote yourself by drinking coffee or by applying a camphor rub to yourself.

What if you generally feel better and your chronic complaint is improving, but you also develop a few strange new symptoms that you never had before? If these new complaints last only a few days, it is a sign that a good remedy has been chosen — but that you are temporarily developing additional symptoms that can be caused by the remedy. This outcome means that the remedy will give you significant help, but may not be your true simillimum. However, if these symptoms persist and become much worse, the remedy was incorrect. Your homeopath may ask you to antidote the remedy and will then prescribe a new one.

Finally, don't forget that remedy reactions include mental, emotional, and behavioral symptoms as well as physical ones. In my own experience, I have found that remedies can bring up emotional wounds from the past — feelings of grief, insecurity, anger, and jealousy. Sometimes, these experiences can be rather embarrassing, because they make you much more acutely aware of your own emotions and behavior. It is as if you were watching yourself from a more objective perspective and becoming more aware of your flaws. Please try to stick with these experiences and not run away from them. By becoming more aware of a problem, you can also overcome it. Time and time again, I have seen how a correct remedy can provide this kind of information to patients, and how they eventually find healing as a result.

FOLLOW-UP VISITS

When treating cases of chronic disease, most homeopaths ask patients to return for a follow-up appointment after four to six weeks. The reason is that it usually takes about a month to assess the effects of a prescribed remedy. Obviously, in acute cases (for example, ear infections, the flu, asthmatic crises, etc.), remedy response is evaluated much more quickly, usually within hours or even minutes. Follow-up visits are usually a half hour in length, although this may vary depending on the situation. Some homeopaths will take follow-up consultations by phone, especially in acute cases that need to be monitored on a more frequent basis.

During a follow-up visit, it is critical that you supply your homeopath with complete details about your remedy response. This information will be used to determine whether or not treatment was successful, as well as how to proceed. Your homeopath will be particularly interested in the following information:

• *Your general health response.* Any positive or negative changes in mental state; feelings of well-being; vitality; and general body functions such as appetite, sleep, dreams, menstruation, bowel function, sexual desire, etc.

• *The progress of your primary complaint.* This includes patterns of symptom improvement or worsening over time.

• *The appearance, severity, and longevity of new symptoms.* These may include complaints from the past that have now returned, or completely new complaints. You should also report any reactions such as rashes, diarrhea, vomiting, or nasal discharge.

• *Emotional, mental, and behavioral responses.* These include positive or negative trends in relationships, at work, and in your emotional and mental state.

Obviously, to provide good feedback to your homeopath, some self-observation and record-keeping can be useful. It is always a good idea to jot down a few notes before each appointment. However, don't go overboard; a general outline of trends and events is sufficient.

Depending on your remedy response, your homeopath will make a decision about what to do next. If your response has been good, or if there has been at least some improvement without relapse, your homeopath will most likely decide to wait and not redose. As stated earlier, once a healing reaction has been set into motion, it is best not to tamper with it unless there has been a definite relapse. So don't be disappointed if your homeopath decides not to give you any more remedy at your follow-up. It means that they believe your situation will continue to improve further, without additional aid.

On the other hand, if your homeopath feels that their remedy selection was correct but your vital force needs another nudge toward health, they will probably suggest another dose of the same remedy. This dose may be of the same, higher, or lower potency. If you are on liquid dosing, your homeopath may simply ask you to continue what you are doing, or they may alter your dosing slightly.

If your case is not progressing, your homeopath will probably decide to analyze your case further and try a new remedy. If several remedies have been tried unsuccessfully over a period of time or have had only minor ameliorative effects, your homeopath may start from scratch with a new intake interview. This will provide both of you with the opportunity to rethink things, and for you to provide new information that you may have forgotten or withheld. Of course, you should feel free to tell your homeopath new information at any appointment.

Like all health care practitioners, homeopaths will, on occasion, decide to consult with colleagues on difficult cases. Sometimes they may refer you to another practitioner who they feel might have better insight into your case. If you feel your health is not improving as it should, you should also feel free to consult with another homeopath on your own. As mentioned earlier, it is important that your relationship with your homeopath be open and free-flowing. If you cannot discuss your case with them or if they cannot effectively make use of the information you provide, their ability to find a good remedy for you will be limited.

WHEN TO REPORT BACK TO YOUR HOMEOPATH

As with any kind of doctor or healer, if you have a question for your homeopath or if a crisis arises, please call them. Most homeopaths have answering services or other means of responding quickly to their patients. In the course of chronic treatment, it is appropriate and even preferable that you call your homeopath when an acute ailment arises, rather than try to deal with it on your own. Most homeopaths prefer to treat problems that arise with simple and natural methods (bed rest, fluids, etc.) or with remedies, rather than have patients suppress their symptoms with cold medicines, nasal sprays, painkillers, or even antibiotics. For example, if you are being treated for arthritis and you develop the flu, call your homeopath. Don't forget, homeopathy is holistic medicine. The problem you are experiencing may seem unrelated to your chronic complaint, but in reality, all of your symptoms are part of your overall health picture.

MIXING HOMEOPATHY WITH OTHER TYPES OF TREATMENT

This brings us to an important question: how does homeopathic treatment interact with allopathic or other types of alternative treatment? Is it all right to pursue other forms of treatment and to use homeopathy as well? The answer to this is yes — and no.

Ideally, it is preferable not to mix medical treatments. If you are seeing a homeopath, an acupuncturist, an herbalist, and an allopath, and you are regularly taking over-the-counter medicines, vitamins, and herbs, how will your homeopath be able to accurately assess the effects of your treatment? Was your remedy antidoted by all of these other things you are doing? Was your response to a remedy immediately suppressed or altered? Unfortunately, it has become increasingly common for people to try many different kinds of healing modalities at the same time. This may seem to buy relief, but to a practitioner, it only brings confusion. How will you yourself know what is really helping you, or if one of your many treatments is actually causing harm?

That said, some types of treatment do cause less interference with homeopathy than others. In my experience, noninvasive body therapies such as massage, craniosacral therapy, and osteopathic treatment do not interfere with homeopathic treatment. Chiropractic treatment is also usually noninterfering. Passive forms of energy healing such as Reiki and prayer also blend effectively with homeopathy, and can even boost its effects. In contrast, using homeopathy alongside other aggressive forms of energy medicine such as acupuncture can be trickier; one must be careful to have such treatments work synergistically, not in opposition to one another.

Personally, I have become increasingly conservative about my use of all forms of medical treatment. I used to take many daily vitamins and would think nothing of trying out all kinds of herbal supplements. Today, I am extremely judicious about what I put into my body and what treatments I undergo. Now that I have trained in homeopathy for several years, I am all too aware that everything we do, eat, and drink can have effects.

Of course, I also believe that my body is strong enough to withstand most things. I don't worry about minor lapses here and there, nor am I obsessive about dietary restrictions. People often ask me, "What is the homeopathic dietary recommendation?" My answer is always, "Nothing in particular. Just eat a balanced diet." Homeopathic lifestyle recommendations simply call for the maintenance of good hygiene and the avoidance of obviously egregious practices such as heavy smoking, excessive alcohol and coffee drinking, and extremes in drug or junk food intake — good common sense and moderation.

So what about allopathic treatment? Of course, there are situations where allopathic treatment cannot be discontinued or avoided. Certainly, allopathy is a must in the case of a serious accident or when surgery is required. Similarly, diabetics must stay on their insulin; severe asthmatics and those with extreme blood pressure problems cannot go off their medications; and those who have taken steroids, hormones, or antidepressants for a long time cannot stop "cold turkey."

Luckily, homeopathy can usually work alongside allopathic treatment. The use of daily liquid dosing or more frequent low-potency dry-dosing can help keep the vital force stimulated, even if allopathic medicines are having antidotal effects. And, as mentioned earlier, the closer a remedy is to a patient's simillimum, the more likely that it will work through any other treatment.

But it is always preferable to take less medicine than more, if it can be managed safely. With patience and an ever-strengthening vital force, a patient undergoing homeopathic treatment will often be able to slowly wean herself off allopathic medicines. Thus, asthmatics may be able to gradually decrease their use of inhalers, and psychiatric patients may be able to decrease the frequency and amount of their medications. I even know of severe arthritics who have been able to withdraw from their daily intake of steroids and painkillers and find lasting cure with homeopathy. Such cures take time, commitment, expert homeopathic care, and collaboration with a patient's allopath to make sure that withdrawal is conducted in a safe and effective manner. But these kinds of cures do happen.

But what if complete cure isn't possible? It has been my experience that in situations where patient health has been too compromised for complete cure, homeopathy can at least bring relief and a greater sense of vitality. My own mother, now in her late 80s, still takes all of her allopathic medications. But ever since she began to see a homeopath a few years ago, she has had greater energy and vitality. I truly believe it has given her a new lease on life.

What about vaccination? Each parent or patient must decide for themselves what to do about this difficult issue. I have already discussed at length the damaging effects that mass vaccination programs can have and their potential role in the increase of chronic disease today. Vaccination is also counterproductive to effective homeopathic treatment. But there *are* homeopathic methods for treating the negative effects of vaccines. And there are also homeopathic approaches to treating and preventing the diseases that vaccinations are used to prevent. My advice is to educate yourself as best as you can and make your own decision; don't let others make it for you. Many web sites provide excellent alternative information about vaccination. A few places to start are *www.healthy.net/vaccine, www.909shot.com,* and *www.nccn.net/~wwithin/vaccine.htm.* The reading list provided at the end of this book includes several informative books about vaccination as well.

Finally, there is the problem of self-medicating. One of the greatest challenges that today's homeopathic patients face is learning not to run to the drugstore and suppress every acute ailment that crops up. Even if someone is dedicated to giving homeopathy a try, it may take a bit of time for them to discover that they can survive a cold without cold medicine, a cough without cough syrup, an ear infection without antibiotics, a rash without cortisone, and a fever or headache without aspirin. Frankly, it took me a couple of years to finally make the break and stop these almost instinctual responses to minor ailments. However, it can be done. Half the time you can ride through minor problems with good old-fashioned bed rest, lots of fluids, and some efforts at removing stress from your life. The rest of the time, homeopathy can come to the rescue and get you through. But don't be worried if you do need to resort to allopathy now and then. Every person must find the road to recovery that they are most comfortable with and that works for them.

STICK WITH IT!

At the end of Chapter 3, I spoke about the importance of attitude and informed participation in the homeopathic healing process. Homeopathy is not always a quick fix. This is especially true in cases of chronic disease. If your allopath hasn't been able to cure you with many years of treatment, why should a homeopath be able to cure you overnight? True healing takes time and dedication. It may also involve some ups and downs. Your health is at stake, and it's worth it.

Effective homeopathic treatment will also demand that you dig deep, examine your life, and engage openly and honestly with your homeopath. How can you find a cure if you are not willing to let your homeopath know what is really going on? There is no medical instrument for determining the nature of your vital force. It can only be determined through what you disclose to your homeopath. So, be an involved and optimistic patient. Seek a second opinion when necessary. Ask for more information and explanations when uncertain. Do not hold back on information, and keep your eye on the goal — true cure.

That's really what this book is all about — enabling you to recognize the extraordinary healing power of homeopathy and find it for yourself.

CHAPTER 9

⌘

CURE *IS* POSSIBLE

"Conventional medicine conveniently dismisses... stories as 'anecdotes' — but I recall a wonderful tale about Steven Hawking, the theoretical physicist... Evidently one of his graduate students had just penetrated the notion that all these little subatomic particles didn't have a material presence in the Newtonian billiard-ball sense at all, but were rather transient arrangements of energy... Lost in his disorientation... [he] asked Hawking what held the universe together. Hawking leaned back in his wheelchair and said, 'Stories.'"

— WILL TAYLOR, MD, 1997 [WT4]

THIS CHAPTER IS FULL OF CURE STORIES, MANY OF THEM WRITTEN in the words of a patient or family member directly touched by the miracle of homeopathy. You've read my own amazing story about Max's cure. In the world of homeopathy, anecdotes like these are almost commonplace. Indeed, most homeopaths decide to practice homeopathy because they have undergone a "conversion" experience — a cure that touched them and left them forever changed. Will Taylor, MD, the homeopath whose words introduce this chapter, experienced the cure of an intractable case of shingles. As he writes:

"My first formal training in homeopathy was the IFH [International Foundation for Homeopathy] professionals course. We were all formally-trained allopathic doctors and nurses and such. The first class we went around the room and told how we'd come to be interested in homeopathy. Nobody was there because of a theoretical convincement. Each person had an 'anecdote' to relate — my desperate and wonderfully successful consultation of a 'quack' to treat my shingles, an MD mom with a kid successfully rescued from dialysis and impending kidney transplant by a single dose of *Apis* [made from honeybee poison], lots of Arnica stories (sometimes I wonder if God gave us the Arnica plant to entice us into homeopathy). I don't think there was a dry eye in the room at the end of the session...

This is an empirical science. Galileo did not get far trying to reason with people as to why there might be moons around Jupiter. He asked them to look in the telescope... I would ask any skeptic, just as Galileo did, 'Please just look. It's there.' Homeopathy does not fit into the worldview I held before my shingles were cured, and it will never fit into that worldview, just as Galileo's moons will never fit into the pre-Galileon views of the universe. Homeopathy has changed my view of the world and how it works. Don't deny yourself the opportunity to expand your view as well. Please just look in the telescope." [WT4]

As it turns out, many of the world's greatest homeopaths started off as skeptical allopaths who later became ardent supporters of homeopathy once they experienced its power. In Chapter 4, I related the story of Constantine Hering, MD, the father of American homeopathy, who first approached homeopathy as a debunker. Another former skeptic became one of the greats of British homeopathy, James Compton Burnett, MD. Burnett attended medical school in Vienna in 1865 and was awarded the Gold Medal in Anatomy upon graduation. The last thing on his mind at the time was homeopathy. As reported in a biography of Burnett published by John Henry Clarke, MD, in 1904:

"Burnett left University with strictly orthodox medical views, 'having been taught by good men and true that Homoeopathy was therapeutic nihilism.' This was the current view at the time, often expressed with a great deal more virulence. Homoeopathy in Britain was confined to a more or less persecuted sect, actively ridiculed in the universities...

While working at a hospital, Burnett watched a little boy die of pleurisy. It affected him greatly. He confided his despondency to his friend Alfred Hawkes at the Royal Infirmary, who recommended homeopathy. Dr. Burnett purchased — 'very much as if I were con-

templating a crime' — Richard Hughes's two manuals... which at that
time provided the standard introduction in English to 'this dangerous
ground.'

Said Burnett, 'I mastered their main points in a week or two, and
came from a consideration of these to the conclusion either that
Homoeopathy was a very grand thing indeed, or this Dr. Hughes must
be a very big —. No, the word is unparliamentary. You don't like the
word? Well, I do, it expresses my meaning to a T; on such an important subject there is for me no middle way, it must be either good clear
God's truth, or black lying.'

Hughes had suggested Aconite as a remedy for simple fever and
Dr. Burnett determined to test the advice on his children's fever ward,
dosing all the patients down one side with Aconite and treating the
others as usual. 'Within twenty-four hours all the Aconite children
were cured (save one who had measles) and smartly discharged, while
the rest still languished in hospital. The experiment was repeated with
the same startling results until a truculent nurse, impatient of the doctor's hard heart, dosed all the patients indiscriminately from 'Dr.
Burnett's Fever Bottle' and emptied the ward.'

Burnett said he was 'simply dumbfounded.' He spent his nights
reading homoeopathic literature, and 'having suffered a conversion
which he afterwards compared to St. Paul's on the road to Damascus,
instantly resolved 'to fight the good fight of Homoeopathy with all the
power I possess; were I to do less I should be afraid to die.'" [Clarke]

Burnett went on to write 24 books about homeopathic treatment
and was one of the first to write about vaccines triggering chronic illness. He was also the father of British author Ivy Compton-Burnett, as
well as the great-uncle of Marjorie Blackie, MD, a homeopath who
served as physician to Queen Elizabeth for many years.

In many ways, Burnett's conversion experience was a very modest
demonstration of the power of homeopathy. Striking cures of much more
serious ailments are easy to find, as the rest of the stories in this chapter
will attest. I collected them between 1997 and 2000, largely from con-
tributors to an international homeopathy Internet list. Over the past few
years, I have gotten to know several of these individuals personally.

You will find that the anecdotes in this chapter cover a wide range of diseases. They include supposedly incurable conditions like Alzheimer's disease; serious acute situations like heart attack, kidney failure, coma, and hemorrhage; and chronic conditions like depression, migraine, and fibromyalgia. But even the smallest of cures is a miracle when it flies in the face of everything we have been taught by the allopathic world. I hope that you will find these stories to be powerful food for thought and an inspiration to explore the world of homeopathy for yourself.

ALZHEIMER'S DISEASE REVERSED

At one of my homeopathic training seminars I witnessed videos of a woman cured of Alzheimer's disease. The changes in her over the course of several months of treatment were nothing short of miraculous. I have heard of other cases of successful Alzheimer's disease treatment as well. One is the story presented below — one of the most impressive tales of homeopathic healing I have ever read. It is written by the daughter of a man whose Alzheimer's disease went into remission for several years thanks to homeopathic treatment:

> "I've had a request that I repost my story about my Dad and Alzheimer's... It's not a medical paper. It's just a story... a story with a happy ending. This story was written over a year ago. In July, it will be two years since his first dose [of the remedy]. My Dad continues to do well. He is now off all other medications. He can drive in town. He rewired a lamp the other day! And he's helping my Mother replace a bad bios chip on her motherboard. He's not perfect, but he's not curled in a ball on the floor in the fetal position."

Original posting:

> "I want all of you with loved ones suffering from Alzheimer's disease to know that I understand what you and your families are experiencing. My father has been diagnosed with Alzheimer's disease for over a year now. My mother had been dropping hints that something was seriously wrong for quite some time when we spoke almost daily on the phone. But nothing that she told me prepared me for what I found when I visited home in July of this year.

The Dad that I knew was no longer there. He knew me, but did not know my husband. He slept most of the day and night. When awake he was either hostile and combative, or curled into a defensive posture. His paranoia was constant. He thought everyone was trying to poison him through his food and medicine. He thought everyone was making fun of him. He had no short term memory. He resented my mother, yet she was the only one he trusted. He had tuned out — he didn't know his address, what year it was, who was president. He was having vivid, violent dreams. He was exhibiting some bizarre behaviors like stashing bags of paper trash all over the house and outbuildings. These were just a few of the symptoms. I'm sure you know the profile.

I was devastated. I came home paralyzed. I thought, 'How can my mother handle this? How can we afford full-time care?' I couldn't sleep or eat. I was worried about my father, my mother, and the rest of our family. My husband and friends immediately set about looking into therapies for Alzheimer's disease. My husband would come home with a score of papers, references, books, and other information. I couldn't listen to them, I just couldn't read anything. What little I did hear or read, I knew my parents would not be willing to try. There were a lot of radical and sometimes invasive therapies suggested. Therapies that were not available near my parents. Therapies that I knew my mother would not want.

Suddenly, I remembered my mother telling me that when you've got a problem, you first do everything you know how to do, and then when you've exhausted your knowledge and ability, you turn to God and say, 'Lord, I've done all that I know how to do, tell me what to do.' I decided to use a therapy that I knew worked — something that I knew how to do. I decided to use a therapy that I had been using successfully for years on myself and my family.

I called my homeopathic physician, Dr. Jennifer Smith. Dr. Smith is a naturopathic physician who specializes in homeopathy. She recently moved from my area to Denver to do research on homeopathic treatment... Dr. Smith... gave me a long list of questions to ask my mother about my father — everything from his eating habits to his dreams. I am grateful that my mother is such an observant caregiver. It took a couple of hours on the phone to get the answers I needed because my father would walk through the room and wonder why my mother was talking about him. The paranoia again. I then called Dr.

Smith and let her run through the questions and I answered them. It took about an hour on the phone with her. Dr. Smith then recommended a homeopathic remedy...

Dr. Smith said that we might notice a slight difference in my father in three or four weeks. However, it took my mother two days to get my father to take the remedy. He thought we were trying to poison him. He did eventually take it. It was one tiny little $\frac{1}{16}$ inch tablet dissolved under the tongue. [Dr. Smith] said he may never have to take it again, or he may need a repeat dose. She was not sure, we'd have to wait and see and be very watchful.

He took the remedy on a Tuesday or a Wednesday... I talked to my mother Friday, and she said, 'Well, your father participated in a conversation at the restaurant this morning after church. He hasn't done that in a couple of years. Interesting, huh? Let's see what happens.'

Well, by Saturday, *all of his symptoms had reversed*. Memory problems, *gone*. Paranoia, *gone*. Inability to solve problems, *gone*. The feeling that he had been betrayed by everyone, *gone*. All of his symptoms were *gone*. By Sunday (four days after taking the remedy) he was making witty and sarcastic jokes on the phone in the background while I was talking to my mother on the phone. My mother says that he is better than he has been in 20 years. On the Saturday after taking the remedy, he installed a window air conditioner for some friends of ours. On the following Wednesday, the power had gone out at the house. The village said the power would not be back on for a couple of hours. My mother was holding her ceramics class in her shop. My father hotfooted it out to the garage and hooked up the house to a generator!

The changes in my father have been *so* significant, that everyone in town has noticed and cannot believe the difference. Just by chance, my parents both had their six-month doctor's appointments the week before last. The doctor saw my mother first and remarked, 'Mary, what's up? I haven't seen your blood pressure this low in years!' Mother responded by showing him the bottle that the remedy came in. She said, 'See this. This is why my blood pressure is so low. I didn't take it, Ernie (my father) did. And I want you to know that the shipping to get the remedy here cost more than the remedy itself.' The doctor finished with my mother and went with her across the hall.

Now, I want you to know that this was a man who on his last doctor's visit did not know his name, what year it was, or who was President.

When they walked in the door, my dad was sitting there reading *Time Magazine*. He looked up and said, 'Hey, do you guys realize that our Dodge minivan has been recalled? The back door could pop open at any time!'... The doctor was shocked. By this time my mother was standing behind Dad and gave the doctor a shrug of her shoulders. He just couldn't believe it! As a matter of fact, the doctor is anxious to know more, and we're going to have him contact my homeopathic doctor.

When my mother discussed it with her doctor, and when I discussed it with my homeopathic doctor, we all remarked that so many people could be helped by this. Thousands and thousands of Alzheimer's patients and caregivers could be helped. All those lives could be changed for the better even if there were a moderate improvement in symptoms.

People don't often turn to alternative medicine until they're desperate. But, I know from my own family's experience, that there is no one more desperate than the caregiver of an Alzheimer's patient. It is truly worth a try. The treatment was easy. It was noninvasive. There were not elaborate regimes to follow. There was only a few hours of our time and one little tablet taken one time. The whole therapy including the remedy, long distance phone charges, and consultation fees came to less than $100. It is truly the best money I've ever spent. Everyone would not react so quickly and have as dramatic a result as my father; but even if symptoms were lessened, many lives could be improved." [MW]

CANCER CURES AND EXPULSION OF TUMORS

In Chapter 6, I mentioned the extensive work on cancer treatment going on in India. Indian homeopaths like Dr. A. U. Ramakrishnan of Madras and Dr. Pradip Banerji of Calcutta have successfully treated hundreds of patients with cancers of many forms, including cancers of the brain, lung, breast, cervix, ovary, pancreas, prostate, rectum, skin, bone, and leukemia. For example, between 1993 and 2000, Dr. Ramakrishnan treated 170 cases of rectal cancer, 66 of which he considered to be viable for homeopathic treatment. He claimed success in 54 of these cases [Ramakrishnan].

Of course, cancer was around back in the 1800s as well. Several homeopaths of the late 19th century were well-known for their cancer cures, including Irish homeopath Robert Cooper, MD, and James Compton

Burnett, MD, the British homeopath whose conversion story was described earlier. But once the allopathic establishment took over in the United States, the use of homeopathy for cancer — indeed, the use of anything else besides surgery, radiation, or chemotherapy — was legally prohibited. Nevertheless, one 20th-century American homeopath was also known for his cancer cures — Arthur Hill Grimmer, MD. Between 1925 and 1929, one hundred fifty biopsy-diagnosed cancers were reputedly cured by his treatment with homeopathy [Winston, p. 299].

Among the many interesting cancer-related stories found in the old homeopathic journals is the following one published in a letter to *The Homoeopathic World* in 1924 by Canon Roland Upcher, a clergyman from Norfolk, England, who also functioned as a lay homeopath. It illustrates how homeopathic remedies can get the body to expel foreign or harmful materials — in this case, a tumor. Whether or not the tumor in this case was actually cancerous we will never know, but homeopathic treatment did have the necessary effect. The story also touches upon the role of vaccination as a causative factor in disease:

"A woman, fifty years of age, was taken into a certain hospital in a former parish of mine — suffering from great pain in the lower abdomen with vomiting, she was unable to keep any food down. Two eminent surgeons... met the three local practitioners in consultation. They unanimously diagnosed the case as undoubtedly cancer... The X ray was not used. But as it was in so difficult a position it was judged too dangerous to operate upon; and the poor woman was sent home to die... The woman was in such a desperate condition, that she could only lie in bed and groan. She neither could take any food nor retain nor pass anything. Under these circumstances, I determined to see whether Homoeopathy could do any good.

First Question: 'Have you any history of consumption [tuberculosis] in your family?'
Answer: 'Yes! My brother and sister both died of consumption.'
Second Question: 'Have you ever been revaccinated?'
Answer: 'Yes; about five years ago, and I have never been well since.'
Third Question: 'Did you ever have a bad fall, or blow in your stomach?'...

Answer: 'Yes; when I was about seventeen or eighteen, I fell off a swing on to my stomach.'

Now follows the treatment according to Homoeopathy. In the first place I had to knock down two stone walls before the indicated remedy could get through to the local mischief. The first wall was that of Consumption. Received five globules of Bacillinum 20 [a nosode of tuberculosis] in single dose. Called three days afterwards, found the woman gone out, had walked a mile and a half down to the town. Next day... I called again.

'Well, Mrs. F., are you mad? What have you been doing, going walking to town?'

Answer: 'Well, sir, I felt, and still feel, so much better; I can eat and drink and keep it down, and I have less pain.'

Wall No. 1 knocked down. Next came the Vaccinal wall and she received two doses, one drop of Thuja (mother tincture), twenty-four hours apart. [*Thuja*, made from Eastern white cedar, is a remedy known for counteracting vaccination damage.] Called at the end of the week. The woman met me at the door with 'Please, sir, a discharge has set in!' 'Good gracious! Where from?' 'Please, sir, from the womb!'

This discharge continued for a week and the tumour in the abdomen, with outside swelling nearly as big as a football, slowly subsided. But as the woman appeared so weak and prostrate with the discharge, I got frightened and judged it well to antidote the Thuja, so administered Pulsatilla 30c, one dose. Next day the discharge decreased and the tumour immediately began to swell up again. Question: Is Wall No. 2 knocked down? Cannot tell, but anyhow the woman is a 'Daisy': so I will try the Homoeopathic rule and give her some 'Daisy.' Anyhow, it is God's remedy for bruises...

[In other words, Upcher determined that the remedy that matched this woman was *Bellis Perennis*, made from daisy. It also happens to be a good remedy for bruises and injuries; recall, she had a fall from a swing onto her stomach.]

She accordingly received three drops of Bellis Perennis (mother tincture), and I left her with the remark, 'I think you will find that will do your belly good!' Unable to visit again for a week. When I had to go into the woman's neighbourhood... called, found the woman washing clothes in back kitchen. 'Well, how are you, Mrs. F.?' 'Quite well thank you, sir!' 'Quite well?!! How's that?' 'Well, sir, three days after you gave me that last dose, I had a great bearing down as if I was going to have a baby and THAT thing all came away, four pounds of it, and I and my husband buried it in our garden!'

Reflection. The two stone walls having been knocked down by Bacillinum and Thuja, Bellis was able to get through and do its work." [Upcher]

MORE EXPULSION ANECDOTES

There are many other fascinating expulsion stories to be found in the homeopathic literature. I have already mentioned the story of a dental hygienist who, after homeopathic treatment, passed visible quantities of mercury in her menstrual blood. Here are three more anecdotes, one describing the expulsion of a long-forgotten piece of glass embedded in a man's leg (also with Bellis Perennis); another, the purging of arsenic; and the last, painless passage of a kidney stone.

Glass Be Gone

"On Labor Day, 1992, my friend Lester had to leap through a second story window to save his life from a fire. He landed partially in the tree in the front yard, and had a fractured tibia among other things. I gave him some remedies at that time. He then moved two hours away, inasmuch as his home was destroyed and he needed a place quickly.

Last year, in October 1994, after Lester had moved back into the city, he complained of pain in his left leg on the outer side, a few inches above the ankle. I gave him one pellet of Ruta 200c. He said he felt immediate relief. (At this time I was working on the assumption that it must be a ligament.) [*Ruta Graveolens*, made from rue, is often used for ligament pain and strain.]

About December 1994, he told me that his leg was again bothering him. He described it as "It feels like a piece of bone is coming out," which I dismissed because it had been two years since the fire, and he was walking. However, he often limped. I gave him one pellet of Ruta 1M and he said he felt something happening, but couldn't describe it well, although he said it always felt better after a remedy.

In February 1995, Lester was visiting and began limping again. I began to think he had a very deep injury to the periosteum, which led me to a remedy that Dr. Subrata K. Banerjea spoke of during a seminar I attended. Dr. Banerjea, of India, told us he had included ancestral tips from his grandfather and father when authoring his Materia Medica. Dr. Banerjea's tip: 'Bellis Perennis: Sprains and bruises, myalgias and neuralgias, rheumatism, boils, etc. Potency 50M. Ancestral tip: Complaints resulting from injuries to deeper tissues and nerves. Potency par excellence!'

I gave the suggested remedy in the suggested potency — Bellis Perennis 50M [Daisy diluted to the degree of $100^{50,000}$] — to my friend at about 10 P.M. on a Wednesday night. On Friday morning he called me to say 'Around 2 A.M. (Friday morning) I woke up and felt something strange going on with my leg, I felt something moving and poking out of my skin. I was sure it was bone. I took the courage to pull it out of my leg. It came out effortlessly. It had only two drops of blood on it. There was no oozing, pus, or anything and the skin sealed up by 9 A.M. that morning. The thing was two inches long and one inch wide and covered with bloody goo. It looked like a bone. I decided to wash it off and keep it. After washing it, I discovered it was a shard of glass, obviously from the bedroom window I jumped out of. I took medicines all my childhood life, and I never had anything work that quickly.'

When I saw the piece of glass I was truly amazed. Little did I imagine that this was an old wound with a foreign object in it. One end of the glass is pointy (the end which was poking out of his skin), but the other end looks like it broke off... Lester walks normally and also dances again. He is totally convinced of the miracle of Homoeopathy." [Maiolino]

Sweating Arsenic

"In 1932, it was my privilege to study under Sir John Weir of London, England,... the Royal Physician, and one of the leading homoeopaths of that time. During one of his lectures, he told us that a single dose of 1M to 10M of the specific substance that was causing the symptoms would allow the body to expel the offending material quickly and easily.

My first experience with this principle was in 1936, just after my return from four years of missionary work in Africa. A 42-year-old orchardist staggered into my office and collapsed on the couch in the waiting room. He was cyanotic; he was perspiring profusely; and his pulse was too rapid to count. 'Doc,' he said, 'I'm dying.' I was inclined to agree with him! As an apple grower, he had many small exposures to arsenic over the past 20 years. While working inside a spray tank, he finally received sufficient additional exposure to throw him into an acute toxic condition. Knowing he would never live long enough to make it to the hospital, I stood next to him feeling quite helpless. Suddenly I recalled the lessons of Sir John Weir. From some remedies brought back from London, I found a 10M potency of Arsenic [arsenic trioxide diluted to the degree of $100^{10,000}$], and poured a half a teaspoon of these granules on his tongue.

Within an hour, his pulse began to slow down but he still perspired freely. An hour later I was startled to hear him call me. Arriving quickly at his side, he pointed to a white powder that was appearing where the perspiration was drying on the folds of his blue shirt. As he brushed it off, he smelled it and then tasted it. 'This is white arsenic, Doc,' he said. 'There is enough here to kill three men!'

It seems the one dose of homoeopathic arsenic changed the body's polarity enough so that the toxic arsenic which had been attracted to the cells was now being expelled. Within three hours the patient was able to drive home and was soon completely recovered. He lived the next 41 years of his life free of any further episodes of arsenic toxicity.

I recall this experience to illustrate a simple and practical law of healing. If you know what poison or toxic substance is causing the illness and give a high potency preparation of that substance, you will enable the body to cure itself. This applies to lead, copper, mercury, aluminum, poison ivy, ragweed, and many other substances to which the human body may react in a toxic manner." [Wilson]

Birthing Kidney Stones

"Every once in a while, I have to sit back and give thanks for small pleasures. This morning my husband woke up in great pain... one we have come to recognize as a kidney stone. This makes number five. The first was removed by lithotripsy to the tune of $20,000 ten years ago. It took two tries and caused terrible side effects. We knew at that time, there were at least two stones left behind. These last three stones were identical as far as symptoms, and as with the others, *Berberis* [made from barberry, a plant] saved the day. Forty-five minutes after the remedy was taken, my husband was completely free of pain. He passed the stone eight hours later... with no pain.

It's a frantic moment when your loved one is in such agony. They want something fast and we have to work under pressure. Homeopathy saves the day with a remedy that materially costs near to nothing." [CG]

SOME SERIOUS ACUTES

Some of the stories you have already read give testimony to the utility of homeopathy in emergencies. While I would certainly run to the hospital in a life-or-death situation, there is still plenty of room for homeopathy to help as well. Below are a few testimonials that show how homeopathy can cure in even the most dire and life-threatening situations.

I'll begin with an anecdote from homeopath David Little who practices homeopathy in remote areas of India and Nepal. In this case, he used homeopathy to treat a severe hemorrhage:

"In Nepal I once was called to treat a hemorrhage during an emergency. Now in this case, I did not know the cause of the problem but feared the worst scenario. The flow was profuse red and her limbs were cold and her face was pale. She seemed emotionally upset by talking. I was preparing to take the person to the hospital when I gave her a one teaspoon dose of *Cinnamonium* 200c [made from cinnamon] in medicinal solution. The effect was immediate and dramatic. The woman felt very much better and calmed right down and started talking normally. I wanted to know the cause of the hemorrhage so I suggested that the individual get a complete medical checkup at a hospital. I do not like functioning in the dark.

As she felt so good on the remedy... she did not follow my instructions until she flew back to Europe a few weeks later. On going for a checkup it was found that she had an ectopic pregnancy in which the tube had burst. The ruptured tube and the surrounding area were all healing nicely so they just left things alone. They said they had never seen anything like it before. They wondered how she survived such an incident without surgical intervention and had healed so dramatically instead. She mentioned the homoeopathy, but they acted as if they did not hear her. They would rather consider it a freak of nature then a cure." [DL1]

Here's a story from New Zealand homeopath John Summerville describing his use of *Cactus Grandiflora* (a well-known heart remedy made from night-blooming cereus, a kind of cactus) in a case of heart attack:

> "Years ago my brother-in-law turned up on my doorstep at about 10:30 P.M., walking bent forward, his face ashen and nose quite blue. He was very anxious and complained of not being able to breathe and that he had a massive pain in his back and that it must be out. I also remember lots of eructations [burping]... I could tell immediately that it wasn't a sore back so gave him Cactus 200c and called an ambulance and doctor. By the time the ambulance arrived about five minutes later, he was almost his jokey self. The doc arrived about another five minutes later. My brother-in-law was very nearly back to normal. Doc did his thing and was very doubtful that anything was amiss (he didn't like homeopaths), but reluctantly conceded that perhaps he should go to the hospital just to be on the safe side. Test results a couple of days later showed evidence of a serious heart attack." [JS]

Homeopathy also came to the rescue for British homeopath Francis Treuherz, who was rather obstinate in his refusal to undergo allopathic treatment in a dangerous case of septicemia (blood poisoning) caused by diverticulitis — an infection in a small pocket of the colon lining. While I don't recommend running out of the hospital like Treuherz did, the remedy he used, *Pyrogen* (made from rotten meat and an important remedy for severely septic states) did enable him to recover:

> "I had a strange fever in 1991, collapsed, and was taken to hospital. I was prescribed surgery and intravenous Flagyl with the diagnosis perforated diverticular disease. I had septicemia, peritonitis, a busted gut with walled off omentum, rebound tenderness, and guarding, so I was very weak and feverish.
>
> I refused treatment and they decided to detain me against my will under mental health legislation. But I gave them the slip and staggered out into a cab and went home and took Pyrogen high [in a high

potency]. After an hour I started to stop looking green and was merely gray, says my wife, and then pale. I ate carefully and took a while to recover, with the help of *China* [made from Peruvian bark] also later. That was it." [FT]

In the next story from Australian homeopath Shonit Danwer, a patient whose kidneys had shut down after a car accident was cured by a remedy that matched the causative factor — fright. Both remedies utilized in this case (*Aconite* and *Opium*) are commonly used for ailments caused by frightening situations:

"I had [this] case in the early days of my practice. A patient's urination stopped after he met with an accident, but he had a miraculous escape and had practically no injury, only later to discover that his urination got suppressed. Similarly his kidneys had got shut down. After trying all sorts of modern medicines he was advised to go in for kidney transplant or two-times-a-week dialysis.

He was given Aconite 10M initially and later Opium in different potencies and he was cured in three months 'miraculously'... Aconite is a very good remedy to counter the acute shock state (be it of any type). Then other remedies like Opium can take care of the rest of the case. But always try to individualize the case every time." [SD]

And what about our animal companions? Here's a story about a little dog named Jozey, saved from potentially fatal food poisoning with two low-potency doses of *Pulsatilla*, made from the windflower:

"Jozey got into a box of Valentine's Day chocolate bonbons. She is little and weighs six pounds. She ate about 50 grams of chocolate. I didn't know that chocolate was poison to dogs. She ate it at about 2 P.M., and at 7 P.M., we noticed that she was shaking and relaxing, shaking and relaxing. Then I noticed her abdomen was bloated so much that it was starting to turn black. Her pulse was pounding and hard. I called two veterinary emergency clinics and they both said to bring her in immediately — that it was very serious, and since it had been so long since ingestion, that they could not guarantee that she would even make it through the night since she was now showing signs of heart failure (the heart had to pump so hard to get past the swelling). They also said that even if she did make it through the night, the aftermath of diarrhea might finish her off because she is so little. The starting vet bill would be $300 and go from there. At that point she couldn't walk anymore.

Well, we all went crazy to see our little dog in that state. The kids were crying and so was I, and then it occurred to me to repertorize her case. So I slapped myself sensible and sat down and chose the rubric that had to do with stomach, *"Worse from fats,"* and came up with Pulsatilla. I checked the materia medica. Being a little lap dog (clingy) and not being thirsty by nature [these are characteristics of Pulsatilla], I quickly gave her a Pulsatilla 6x, which brought her around like a miracle!

She got up and started walking around and playing. She let us rub her belly. She started burping. The effect of the remedy lasted one hour. Then she dropped, exhausted. I gave her another dose and then brought her to sleep with me for healing energy, and of course we had a family prayer. Through the night I could hear her burping and burping. In the morning she was back to her old figure again. Her belly had gone from black to pink. She never went into the diarrhea phase. We gave her rice and water for a couple of days and she was fine! Whew! Only two doses of Pulsatilla 6x. Since Pulsatilla turned out to be Jozey's constitutional remedy, it also cleared up her chronic ear infections, coughs, and a skin disorder she had growing on the ends of her ear flaps." [AS]

CHRONIC DISEASE

Much of this book has emphasized the importance of homeopathy in treating chronic disease — disease that allopathy can only palliate or suppress, not truly cure. Below are some additional illustrations of how effective homeopathy can truly be in curing these kinds of ailments — even those cases that have undergone years of ineffective allopathic treatment. I'll begin with a very typical example — a woman who suffered for many years from chronic bladder infections:

"I... had chronic bladder infections to the point of bleeding for about six years, treated with a variety of sulpha drugs — 18 years ago. Doctors I had seen had suggested low doses of antibiotics every day for the rest of my life. What turned me on to Homeopathy was a 1M dose of *Cantharis*. [A common remedy for bladder infections made from Spanish fly.] Literally, the second it was placed on my tongue, the pains and discomfort ceased, and two days later, my E. coli count was so low that the doctor treating me at the time was amazed that I had achieved it without allopathic (conventional) drugs. That sold me on Homeopathy! Since then, I have studied Homeopathy extensively. I have never had a recurrence of cystitis since that dose of Cantharis — over 18 years ago." [MK]

Here's another anecdote of cure from Lyme disease. Over the past few years, homeopathy has become known as an effective treatment for this condition. Cures of Lyme disease have even been reported by the press. For instance, world-famous South African runner Zola Pieterse "who suffered from tick bite fever for over five years, was only cured after seeing a homeopath." [Pieterse] In the story below, the remedy *Ledum* (made from a plant called ledum palustre or marsh tea) came to the rescue:

> "Last summer almost three weeks to the day after returning from a camping trip in Vermont, my husband came down with a flu-like illness, including joint pains, headaches, extreme fatigue, a few other symptoms, and, of course, the bull's eye rash. He went to his doctor who sent him to see the head of epidemiology at a local hospital where he was duly poked and prodded, and inspected (with his permission) by a group of med students. They even photographed the rash for the archives. I guess we don't get too many 'classic cases of Lyme' here in Montreal.
>
> Not liking the sounds of the possible side effects from the antibiotics, he went directly to his homeopath... who prescribed Ledum 1M three days in a row. Each day when my husband took the Ledum, he rallied a little more. At the end of the three days, he seemed fine. A week later, he had what seemed to be a relapse and didn't respond to the Ledum 1M. He was given Ledum 10M. It's been nearly a year now, and he seems to be suffering no further effects from the disease." [LJ]

Here's another story of conversion to homeopathy, in this case of California nurse Sheri Nakken, RN. Her complaint was serious longstanding migraine headaches. Today, Nakken is a homeopath and a well-known antivaccination activist living in Wales, UK. She is also migraine-free:

> "I will tell my story to the skeptics. I had migraines every one, two, or three weeks since 1981. Severe, lasting two days. Tried Chinese medicine including acupuncture/herbs for one year; chiropractic;... rolfing; shiatsu; dietary changes; candida diets and on and on. No results. Also took remedies that I'd buy in the store without seeing a homeopath — no results.
>
> Finally went to a homeopath in Nevada City, California and after two months on one remedy, LM potency, headache free and have been ever since - nearly three years now! No double-blind trial needed for me." [SN]

Nakken goes on to describe how cost-effective her homeopathic treatment was, despite the fact that she initially consulted with a homeopath who was unable to help her:

> "Expensive was having severe migraine headaches... from 1981–1995 — buying ergotamine inhalers for 10+ years at $70 each for migraines; trying Chinese medicine for one and a half years; chiropractic for two years; shiatsu for two years; Nystatin for candida and suffering through those candida diets; missing work and life — all for nothing!
>
> Other than my first bad choice of a homeopath ($500), it only cost me $115 to be totally cured and have migraine symptoms leave (one initial visit $80, remedy $5, follow-up visit $30)!" [SN]

Perhaps the most convincing testimony of homeopathy's efficacy is when allopaths come calling for treatment. In the beginning of this chapter, Will Taylor, MD, described his own conversion to homeopathy after his cure from shingles. Today, Taylor receives many referrals from colleagues in the allopathic community. In the following anecdote, he describes his treatment of a case of Crohn's disease [a chronic and destructive disease of the gastrointestinal tract] — and how the patient's allopath reacted:

> "I get regular referrals from the local MDs. Even got a call from a gastroenterologist one day after a successfully-treated patient saw him in follow-up for Crohn's disease; she'd responded beautifully and had

been asymptomatic for six months. He asked if I was taking new patients. I said sure, and asked if he had a referral for me. He said 'Well, I've got Crohn's.'" [WT5]

HELPING OUR ANIMAL COMPANIONS WITH HOMEOPATHY

As the story of Jozey and the box of chocolates showed, homeopathy provides a cost-effective treatment option for pets. I have found that homeopathic treatment is an especially effective and humane solution for the aging pet. Several years ago, my family spent $5,000 on surgery for our dog who was suffering from pancreatic cancer. It was a rather hopeless situation, and a month or so after her surgery, she became bloated and incapacitated by the daily doses of cortisone that were prescribed for her. When she could no longer move at all, we had to have her euthanized.

A couple of years later, our elderly 17-year-old cat developed hyperthyroidism and the wasting that goes along with it. The vets recommended drugs that would cause her to have chronic diarrhea or, alternatively, surgery and radiation. After our dog's experience, we decided to deal with the situation homeopathically. With the help of remedies and an improved fresh-meat diet, our cat lived for another year, regained her weight, and was symptom-free for all but the last month of her life. In our view, homeopathy provided not only a more cost-effective solution, but a more humane one as well. Here's a similar pet story that underscores the same point.

"Male Himalayan cat 15 years old.

January 1998. I began to notice our cat slowing down. I assumed old age was taking its toll. There was decreased play. When drinking water, he began to scratch the floor automatically with his right paw.

April 1998. He has been getting more confused and spaced-out. He is walking more slowly, with stiffness in his hind quarters. One day he suddenly stopped eating. He would stare at his food and water and attempt to eat, but he couldn't bring himself to do it. He would try very hard, but he would stop, stare at his dish, and then walk away. He would repeat this behavior frequently. He crawled into his bed, stopped grooming, and wouldn't look up. He couldn't seem to focus or respond to stimuli. He could see and hear, but he didn't seem to process any-thing. He had dilated pupils and a dark 'zombie-like' expression. He stopped urinating and had no bowel movements for two days.

The veterinarian couldn't advise any course of treatment and said that the cat would die soon. He reluctantly gave him an intravenous saline solution for dehydration.

I tried *Belladonna* and *Bryonia* simply because it was late at night and they were the closest remedies that I had on hand. He was near death. There was absolutely no response. Then I found one rubric... [that matched]... In the morning I drove an hour to get the only potency [of the chosen remedy] I could get (6x).

Within two minutes of administering the remedy he began to drink water. A few minutes later he began to eat. I repeated the dose in about an hour. He went to his bed and stayed there for the next twelve hours. He barely moved. At the end of twelve hours he had a very large bowel movement. He then began to eat and drink. Over the next two days he resumed his normal eating pattern and began to have clear eyes and a more normal expression.

December 1998. He has now grown quite old. He has had many ups and downs since April. I can see that his life force is quite weak-ened and that sometime soon he will be departing his tired body. I have repeated the remedy when it seemed appropriate. The longest he has gone was six weeks of continual improvement without a relapse. In November, I switched from a liquid dose of 200c to LM1. The improvement was dramatic. He actually began to run and play for a few days as if he were a kitten.

However, that has not lasted. Now I am giving him very tiny amounts of diluted LM2 on a daily basis. It seems to give him some strength and to make him comfortable. He has good days and bad days... Overall the remedy has been wonderful. It has done a remark-able job in prolonging the cat's life and providing him with comfort and more mental clarity as he grows old." [SL2]

FIGHTING STARVATION AND DISEASE IN THE THIRD WORLD

Many of the stories you have read so far attest to the ability of homeo-pathic remedies to improve the body's functioning — for example, enhancing the body's ability to fight infections. Here's an amazing story about homeopath David Little's use of Schuessler's *cell salts* — low-potency remedies made from nutritional mineral salts found in the body — to treat villagers in a poverty-stricken region of Nepal:

"Many years ago a friend of mine in Nepal was treating some very ill people with just the twelve cell salts. He was testing to see how far one could go... The reason for this was that many of the... villagers could use such a simple medicine as an alternative to the crudest, worst allopathy in the world. He told me that these remedies really worked well, although not as deeply nor as successfully as [the full range of] homeopathic remedies. The point was, he could teach a lay person in the village the system in a reasonable amount of time. As I was a homeopath with experience in the Third World, he asked me to help him run a study with him.

I helped him develop his project and taught him the deeper aspects of the materia medica related to nutritional minerals. For several months I... used the twelve cell salts in all cases where it was not too serious to delay [full] homeopathic treatment. I was shocked at how well we did! We treated hundreds of cases in this manner and followed them for months. As this was a study of nutritional minerals, I noted the possible vitamin and mineral deficiencies, and the homeopathic signs of malnutrition... I was amazed to see malnourished children, with many classical signs of malnutrition, protein deficiencies, and low resistance, suddenly begin to show signs of deep healing *without any change in their diet.*

We tried orthodox vitamins and minerals on other children who were ill in general and showed classical signs of deficiency. The supplements made many of these children sick and they could not assimilate them. Supplements made little overall change in most cases, except some of the more gross signs of deficiency. The children on homeopathic nutrition gained weight, strength, vitality, and resistance although they all ate the same diet, lived in the same poverty, under the same poor hygienic conditions. I saw this with my own eyes. I have seen better results with the [full] homeopathic materia medica, but this was done with only twelve mineral remedies by lay persons under my direction.

Such a thing is hard to believe, but I studied this for six months in the worst of conditions in one of the poorest countries on earth... The cost of the twelve cell salts in this study was minimal, the knowledge needed moderate, and the benefit was maximum. Compare this with expensive allopathic medicine and nutritional supplements that have a much more limited therapeutic range. Also compare the side effects and suppression. The number of aggravations was low and only a few cases responded with negative reactions that needed intervention. How did these people on a meager diet of white rice, a little overseasoned dal, and little else, gain strength, health, and recover from many acute and chronic complaints? Remember, we used only twelve cell salts... and we did not specialize in 'nutritional cases'... I treated virulent acute diseases like typhoid, amoebic dysentery, bacillary dysentery, unknown fevers, as well as all the degenerative diseases of the elderly. The quality of life in the young, the chronic, and elderly increased greatly. I did not think such a thing was possible with twelve nutritional mineral remedies in 6x [potency]... This shows just how adaptable the human organism is when given dynamic nutrition. This is not possible with orthodox supplements [traditional vitamins]." [DL2]

Oh, My Aching *#$&(#!

So how about crippling diseases like arthritis or fibromyalgia? Below, homeopath Maria Bohle describes her husband's slow recovery from severe arthritis:

"My husband has been battling with arthritis for many, many years... [He] had some severe knee injuries — including surgery almost 50 years ago. Then came years and years worth of allopathic pain meds — all kinds of prescription stuff. The VA hospital used to give him huge bottles of Motrin, Naprosyn, Indocin and several others. The directions said to take one tablet; he would take three tablets. It culminated in 120 mg of morphine daily given to him by a pain management specialist (it took that much to remove the pain). It was horrible. Franz just kept getting worse, the pain got worse and worse.

Franz also had arthritis everywhere... I don't know if that was the result of all the things he was swallowing for so long or what. He... had cortisone shots in his knees, elbows, shoulders and hands. And had been on massive doses of prednisone for 'inflammatory arthritis.' The allopathic diagnosis was both osteo- and rheumatoid arthritis. His rheumatologist said, 'There is nothing we can do for him.' We finally turned to homeopathy.

At this writing, after four years of homeopathic treatment (and no prescription medicines at all), he now no longer needs to take pain medicines daily. I remember last year when he went a whole day without even taking aspirin — it was a red letter day!! Now we have whole weeks go by without aspirin...

He also had 'trigger thumb,' and one hand was operated on. Three MDs told him when the other thumb started triggering that the only solution was surgery. Wrong. It took a while but that thumb cleared up with homeopathic treatment... And that thumb is now better than the one that had been surgically repaired.

Franz used to have such heat in his thumbs near the base of the hand and in his knees (especially the knees) that it could be felt almost a foot away from the body. All that has cleared up now and it is very rare that he inflames at all, except when walking too far — and that is mechanical damage.

We are not finished, but he is functional and comfortable compared to several years ago. Homeopathy works! But it is not fast! It can be frustratingly tedious. But if my husband continues to improve as much in the next four years as he has in the last four, I will consider it a miracle. But Homeopathy makes miracles — of that I am sure."
[MBohle1]

Another chronic ailment that has become increasingly prevalent is fibromyalgia, an ailment in which soft tissues are constantly aching, supposedly due to a problem with vitamin and mineral absorption. The testimonial below attests to the efficacy of homeopathy in curing years of suffering with this ailment, along with a cure of migraines too:

"I have had fibromyalgia for nearly 18 years. I went through every allopathic test (even in the days when they didn't know what it was) and treatment known to man... I helped form a fibromyalgia support group when there were only four of us present. Now there are eight fibromyalgia support groups in my area with 20 or more members in each. Well, my point is, I've been through it all. I've seen it spread... I meet someone almost every day with it and I tell them to go to a HOMEOPATH!...

I was on vitamin therapy for three years before I realized I wasn't getting better (actually I knew I wasn't better but I was too ill to do anything about it). I was spending four days a week in bed. Then one of my alternative healing doctors found out that studies done on people with fibromyalgia showed that they started to feel better if the minerals were given intravenously. I was terrified of needles, but determined to try anything that might help — I mean I had two small children at home and they had never seen me well. Sure enough... within a week I felt better for the first time. I definitely felt better for the five months that I could afford it... I went for IV therapy twice a week at $100 a pop. I was spending almost $800 a month — out of pocket — for treatment. Unfortunately, every time I stopped the therapy, my fibromyalgia would act up again. Eventually, because of the cost, I had to stop. So I ended up, once again, in constant pain. This was six years ago...

However, three years ago I started going to a homeopath. Within four months my pain was cut in half. By the end of the first year it was cut even more... without even taking a vitamin or mineral (which was great because they always made me nauseated). Now, I only have flare-ups now and then. My migraines went from three a week, to three a month, to three a year. We're still working on that part. But there's definitely been an 80 percent improvement in my health... Nothing works like homeopathy. Nothing." [GE]

THE EMOTIONAL AND BEHAVIORAL REALM

My son Max's story, of course, is testimony to how effective homeopathy can be for chronic mental, behavioral, and emotional problems. I have been contacted by dozens of parents of autistic children who have read articles I have written about his case. Several have tried homeopathy — a few with success. Autism is definitely not an easy condition to cure, but such cures do happen. The following is another testimonial to the effectiveness of homeopathy in the treatment of another "incurable" emotional condition — obsessive-compulsive disorder (OCD):

"I can attest to the power of homeopathy to help children with OCD and its related spectrum disorders (or anxiety disorders in general)...

Many will be able to relate to a child's medical history such as: Prozac for three years, Anafranil for three years, Paxil for two years, Luvox for one year, and Buspar for three years... given to my daughter since she was four years old (10 years total)... and absolutely no cure — not even close. Lots of suppression (thousands and thousands of dollars for meds, blood tests, psychotherapy, etc.), lots of side effects (too many to mention). Yet, a few different homeopathic remedies over the course of a few years and my daughter no longer has the infamous anxiety disorder, OCD, that there is 'no cure' for... The funny thing is... our homeopath treated her for one of her mental symptoms — one that was somewhat unrelated to OCD — and everything else just sort of cleared up. We are going on two years now without any antidepressant or antianxiety meds (which she had been on for 10 years)." [Anon2]

The next case from homeopath Mary Marlowe describes the beautiful recovery of a woman from anxiety disorder. Given a single dose of *Aconite*, a classic remedy for panic and fear made from the monkshood flower, this woman's symptoms slowly abated. Notice how the memory of an exciting cause for her condition was also recovered:

"I had a case about two years ago — a woman, aged 38, with fear in crowds. She had trouble especially at large outdoor gatherings and at the indoor shopping mall, but really any place where there were a lot of people. She could think of no reason for it, and had managed to avoid these situations until she started a family... Her main problem was a feeling of being pushed into other people, because of the crowding, and she found that very disturbing. She would experience panic and would want to leave. If she could not, she felt frantic. She would feel the need to sit down and longed for fresh, cold air. Twice she had fainted in such circumstances.

Her sense of smell was quite acute — she could not stand perfumes or fragrances. She told of smelling natural gas (the marker scent), when no one else could. She followed the smell, and found a neighbor several houses over who had replaced his gas hot water heater the day before... Noises bothered her, especially when she was trying to concentrate. She could not read or talk on the phone when the television or radio was on...

She found herself rising to urinate during the night — usually at 12:30 A.M. and 2:00 A.M.... She got laryngitis, often around the holidays (November/December) and in the spring (March/April). Allergy symptoms — stuffy nose, itchy eyes... Nightmares, with starting from her sleep — heart pounding, sweat soaking the bed. Trouble falling asleep again...

Gave Aconite 30c, to be used the next time she felt panic on going out. She reported six weeks later that she had used it at her husband's company picnic, with immediate relief. Nightmares less frequent, no longer afraid in the dark... Able to go to the mall with the family for trick-or-treating (very crowded, more than usual) without any panic. Still sensitive to smells, but not so bothered by them. Getting up less often to urinate, though still sometimes.

At the four-month follow-up, all symptoms were much better. She remembered that she was involved in an accident when she was 18 months old — she was run over by an automobile in a parking garage after a shopping trip with her mother and grandparents. She was not seriously hurt, but was taken to the hospital. The car ran over her right hand and arm, and there were also tire tracks on the legs of her overalls...

At one year [after treatment], all symptoms were still better. She gets out frequently now, and tells about a street festival she attended with her children... She reports that her allergy symptoms are gone, along with the night sweats, and getting up to urinate. No panic attacks, even in crowds. Also, she is less sensitive to sounds and smells." [MM]

Here's another wonderful recovery story. In this case, a woman with years of depression, menstrual problems, and substance abuse, found far-reaching cure with a single dose of *Aristolochia Clematitis*, a remedy made from the snakeroot plant. In recent years, Aristolochia has emerged as an extremely useful remedy in cases with severe menstrual problems:

"A woman, age 26, came to see me because of severe menstrual problems. She has premenstrual syndrome (PMS) where she feels wretched and weepy. Lots of menstrual pain with a severe dragging down sensation. Brown mucous discharge whenever she has a period. She had an abortion five months previous to my seeing her, which was very devastating emotionally. Her breasts have developed milk six to seven times in the previous three years. History of skin cancers...

After taking the [contraceptive] pill she suffered a huge depression and self-destructive urges. The pill affected her for four years after taking it! She described herself as erratic in everything she does. She gets bored easily and is a big substance abuser — alcohol, dope, cigarettes, coffee. Excessiveness is in her genes, with a family history of addiction.

She is obsessed with death — hangs around graveyards. She never felt there was a point to life... During her childhood, she wanted to be a hermit... She didn't like people and had no friends. She felt the world wasn't real; it seemed two-dimensional. She felt totally isolated and was okay with it. She prayed that aliens would come and take her back. She feels nothing toward other people. If the whole world was demolished tomorrow she wouldn't care. She feels she doesn't belong to the world; things don't affect her. No emotional attachment. She hates consolation and doesn't want anyone to care about her.

I gave her Aristolochia 30c based on the brown discharge during menses, extreme introversion, aggravation from consolation, aggravation from the contraceptive pill (a keynote symptom), mental depression, sensation of isolation, refusal of society, PMS.

Afterwards, she reported feeling really good. Periods went back to normal, discharge disappeared, no PMS, no longer feeling isolated, getting more into life and her work, gave up alcohol altogether, desire for marijuana is disappearing, feeling happier in her relationships. None of these symptoms came back in the years that I knew her." [DK]

MIRACLES HAPPEN

I'll close this chapter with a few more amazing anecdotes. They testify to the kind of power that homeopathic remedies can have when the simillimum is given.

Arnica and Opium Lift Coma

A few years ago, a relative of one of my teachers was in a coma and close to death in a British hospital. The doctors prohibited homeopathic treatment, but family members managed to rub a bit of *Opium* (potentized opium), diluted in water, on his hand. Within minutes he awoke from his coma, spoke to his family congregated around him for about an hour, said his good-byes, and then expired peacefully. Here's another coma story from Gopal Pandey:

> "Thirty minutes after the application of liquid Arnica 30c, the 80+ year-old patient sat up and was ready to go home. He had been knocked off a stationary motor scooter while waiting for a red light... He had been in coma for two days." [GP]

Varicose Veins Heal in Five Minutes

The following story relates a classic rolling back of symptoms with a surprise ending:

> "I just have to relay a miraculous cure that happened in my clinic on Tuesday. This patient is a highly anxious welfare mom who is phobic about being seen in public where she might be criticized, is afraid of losing her health, is claustrophobic, etc. Seven weeks ago she came with a complaint of shortness of breath and lung tightness. I gave her *Argentum Nitricum* [made from silver nitrate, a useful remedy for anxiety]. She said she cried for seven days and then all her lung symptoms disappeared.
>
> The next time I saw her, her lung symptoms remained clear, but all her leg symptoms... came back. One leg actually got run over by a car many years ago and she's had problems with her knee, her leg, and varicose veins ever since. For several reasons I'll skip now, I gave her *Argentum Metallicum* [made from silver]... In five minutes, the gnarly, bulging, very sore varicose veins became taught and pulled into the skin. It's like they almost disappeared! We're talking five minutes for varicose veins which have been pretty horrible for as long as I've been treating this woman (three years) to clear up. I've seen a lot of instant cures in homeopathy, but this one takes the cake — at least for this year." [Anon1]

Facial Scar Tissue Recedes

> "I treated a man with erupting face pustules of 14 years duration. He had seen lots and lots of MDs, and had tried homeopathic treatment from three other practitioners before he came to me. He wore a full face bandage over the beard area to cover the eruptions and scar tissue, gnarled thick and disfiguring...

The remedy I gave was *Syphillinum* [nosode of syphilis] in LM poten-cy. After a dose... the face would erupt with a vengeance over a previ-ously healed eruption, and discharge pus for a week or so... But when the eruption ceased, it left with less swelling and less scar tissue each time. Each bottle of LM remedy brought him to greater and greater improvement of his face... The key is, the scars were disappearing, when eruptions before the remedy left swollen keloidal tissue in their wake." [MBohle2]

Balding and Chronic Fatigue Reversed

"I have been bald since about age 24. All the males on both sides of my family have been bald by about 30, so I think it is safe to assume that my baldness is hereditary. I had an illness that was eventually diag-nosed as CFS [chronic fatigue syndrome] which stopped me from working for nine years. After discovering homeopathy and receiving treatment, I was able to resume work. So what has this got to do with baldness? Since receiving homeopathic treatment my hair is growing back again. It is slowly but surely returning. My family and friends are starting to notice and comment on it. Is it possible for homeopathic treatment to reverse a genetic tendency?" [RM]

In this case, I guess so!

CHAPTER 10

❧

THE ROAD AHEAD

"The Constitution of this Republic should make special provision for Medical Freedom as well as Religious Freedom... To restrict the art of healing to one class of men and deny equal privileges to others will constitute the bastille [prison] of medical science. All such laws are un-American and despotic."

— BENJAMIN RUSH, MD, signer of the Declaration of Independence, late 18th century [Rush]

AFTER READING THE STORIES IN CHAPTER 9, YOU MAY BE EAGER TO go out and find a homeopath. Unfortunately, if you are American, this can be easier said than done. There are simply not enough well-trained homeopaths practicing in the United States. The most fundamental reason for this is also the largest obstacle that homeopathy faces today: its poor legal status.

Since the early 1900s, the practice of medicine in the United States has been governed by state medical practice laws that, for the most part, restrict all forms of healing to licensed practitioners. Unfortunately, there is currently no state that offers licensure for homeopathy as a distinct discipline. Traditional naturopaths, ayurvedic practitioners, Reiki practitioners, aromatherapists, and herbalists are not licensed either. As a result, Americans have a long, uphill road to travel before they can win the medical freedom that founding father Benjamin Rush, MD, thought should be their constitutional right.

LICENSURE VERSUS CERTIFICATION

In order to fully comprehend the issues surrounding legal homeopathic practice, it is important to understand the difference between *certification* and *licensure*. A homeopath is certified if they have obtained a credential that attests to their competency in the practice of homeopathy. A homeopath is licensed if they can practice homeopathy legally in their state.

Ironically, certification and licensure for homeopathy are currently completely independent of one another in the United States. In some states, certain kinds of practitioners may be licensed to practice homeopathy (for example, an MD or a chiropractor may be legally allowed to dispense homeopathic remedies), but their licensing law might not impose any homeopathic certification requirements on them. On the other hand, a practitioner may be certified in homeopathy (for instance, an MD may have the Diplomate in Homeotherapeutics [DHt], or a professional homeopath may be a Certified Classical Homeopath [CCH]), but he or she may not be licensed to practice homeopathy in their state.

As a result of this legal structure, most homeopaths in the United States — even those who are licensed MDs — must treat their patients under a cloud of potential legal prosecution. They might be accused of "practicing medicine without a license" (because they are unlicensed) or their right to practice might be threatened because they are "practicing medicine outside the scope of their license." Given this situation, it is no wonder that there are not many homeopaths to be found in America.

THE FIGHT FOR LEGAL PRACTICE

The net effect of the medical practice laws in most states is a virtual monopoly by allopathy over the practice of medicine. The only way an alternative healing system can become legalized — at least until recently — is for it to create a mini-monopoly of its own, via its own licensing law. That is the path that chiropractors and osteopaths took, and that acupuncturists and naturopathic physicians (who combine naturopathy with some elements of allopathy) are now taking.

Unfortunately, gaining licensure for a profession can be quite expensive — requiring hundreds of thousands, if not millions, of dollars for each state. It also requires a state-by-state professional turf battle, since licensing laws typically restrict the use of practice-specific healing techniques to licensees. For example, acupuncture licensing laws restrict the practice of acupuncture treatments to licensed acupuncturists.

For all of these reasons, licensing efforts require the strong financial backing of thousands of practitioners as well as tremendous political clout — both things that the homeopathic community does not possess at this time. Indeed, many would argue that licensure for homeopathy and many other alternative therapies is inappropriate and unnecessary — because these therapies pose little risk of harm to the public and because their methods of treatment should not be restricted to a particular group.

So what's an aspiring homeopath to do? One option is to obtain a license in an unrelated health care discipline. A homeopath could become an MD, nurse, chiropractor, naturopathic physician, or acupuncturist — as long as that discipline is licensed in their state and its licensing law allows for the practice of homeopathy. For example, there are currently three states that have homeopathic licensing boards for MDs: Arizona (1982), Connecticut (1892), and Nevada (1983).

But how many people are willing to study and become licensed in another discipline just so that they can practice homeopathy? Very few. The sad truth is that, even if an aspiring homeopath becomes an MD, they may still not be able to practice homeopathy legally in their state. Not only will they have spent many years learning a medical system that is philosophically at odds with homeopathy, but in the end, they might be prosecuted for practicing outside the scope of their license. Indeed, the allopathic establishment seems to be particularly antagonistic towards MDs who practice homeopathy. The DHt certification (a certification granted by the American Board of Homeotherapeutics to MDs and DOs) has never been formally recognized by the American Medical Association, despite repeated efforts and broken promises over the past 40 years.

Invariably, the harsh reality of homeopathic practice today is vulnerability and fear. To protect themselves, unlicensed professional homeopaths have their clients sign waivers that clarify the terms and conditions under which they are being treated. They make absolutely clear that they are not licensed physicians and that they do not diagnose or treat any disease per se; rather, they are simply making "recommendations" to improve a patient's overall "well-being." They also will not conduct a physical exam nor dispense remedies. But the truth is, the legality of homeopathy practiced in this way is still tenuous. Clearly, the situation is less than ideal.

NEW HOPE: LEGALIZATION OF UNLICENSED THERAPIES

In the past few years, however, a ray of hope has emerged. Throughout the United States, a new model for medical legislation has emerged: the legalization of unlicensed forms of medicine. It all began in May of 2000, when the state of Minnesota passed groundbreaking legislation — the Complementary and Alternative Health Care Freedom of Access bill, Minnesota Statute 146A. Natural health care advocates in Minnesota managed to devise a new way to legalize unlicensed forms of treatment without resorting to licensure. Their strategy was to fight for the right to *health freedom*. Taking the lead from Benjamin Rush, MD, the activists argued that, just as freedom of access to information depends on freedom of the press, and religious freedom depends on a religious institution's freedom to operate, health freedom depends on a health practitioner's freedom to practice. Thus, if we want to have the freedom to choose our desired form of health care, we must also have legal alternative health care practice.

Minnesota's journey to health freedom began in the mid 1990s, when a popular Minnesota naturopath was prosecuted for practicing medicine without a license, despite the fact that there were no consumer complaints or allegations of harm against her. At the same time, efforts to obtain licensure for naturopathy in Minnesota were failing. Gradually, the natural health community in Minnesota began to realize that working for more licensure laws was not a solution. For one thing, the primary legal purpose of licensing is to protect the public from harmful practices. Since most alternative therapies pose little risk of harm and are not "medicine" in the conventional sense, licensing them is both unwarranted and unnecessary. The Minnesota activists also realized that licensing efforts tend to divide and pit practitioner groups against one another. They wanted to pull together, not pull apart.

In 1997, the Minnesota legislature asked the Department of Health to conduct a study on complementary and alternative medicine (CAM) in Minnesota. The report that emerged laid out a set of guiding principles for handling CAM in that state:

- Consumers should have as broad access as possible to CAM.

- Regulations should be minimized, and should only be imposed to guarantee public safety.

- Explicit legislation was needed to allow providers to practice without fear of prosecution.

The net recommendation of the study was that,

> "Freedom of practice legislation which allows providers to continue service as long as the service is not shown to be dangerous or harmful, should be considered as a possible alternative to licensure or registration when appropriate. This may require making some changes in the Medical Practices Act or other licensure laws." [Minnesota]

Armed with this report, activists garnered widespread public and legislative support. After two years and much hard work, the Health Care Freedom of Access bill was passed. The final bill had several key components:

- Unlicensed practitioners of health care modalities that are deemed unharmful (including naturopathy, homeopathy, massage, and other healing modalities) are exempt from criminal charges of practicing medicine without a license. "Harm" would henceforth be the legal basis for investigations, rather than discrimination against alternative healing methods.

- Unlicensed practitioners could not engage in practices that were not truly "complementary and alternative health care" as defined by the statute. Thus, the practitioners could not perform surgery, dispense controlled substances, puncture the skin, etc.

- A new office in the Department of Health was set up to have jurisdiction over unlicensed practitioners to ensure that they adhere to certain rules of ethical conduct, including prohibitions against fraud, false or misleading advertising, and sexual contact with a client.

Unfortunately, the freedoms won by the new Minnesota legislation did not extend to licensed practitioners who practice alternative medicine. The licensed disciplines would not relinquish full control over their licensees. As a result, those already licensed under the Board of Medical Practice (MDs and DOs), chiropractors, dentists, and podiatrists remained under the jurisdiction of their own licensing boards. When these practitioners engage in CAM, they will still be subject to prosecution for practicing medicine outside the scope of their license.

While not perfect, the Minnesota law provided a precedent for natural health care reform in America. In May of 2002, Rhode Island passed similar legislation. Then, in September 2002, California passed its own health freedom bill, SB-577 — without a single "no" vote from the legislature. I participated in this effort as an executive board member of the California Health Freedom Coalition, the organization that sponsored this bill. The structure of SB-577 differs in a fundamental way from Minnesota's health freedom law: it does not create a new regulatory structure within the state government (and therefore creates no financial burden on the state). Instead, SB-577 simply narrows the scope of the state's Medical Practice Act so that it no longer restricts *all* forms of treatment — only those treatments that create serious risk of harm to the public. Unlicensed practitioners are now free to practice in California, as long as they abstain from certain practices that are reserved for licensed physicians. The new California law also protects patients by imposing disclosure requirements on unlicensed practitioners. Such practitioners are now required to tell clients that they are not licensed physicians, they must explain the rationale behind their method of treatment, and they must disclose their training and experience.

Clearly, the legal climate for homeopathic practice in the United States *is* slowly changing. Health freedom activities are now sweeping across America, with health freedom groups forming and legislative efforts underway in nearly 30 states. Hopefully, Minnesota started a trend that will bring health freedom to all Americans.

HOMEOPATHIC TRAINING

Another critical requirement for the survival and spread of homeopathy is the training of new homeopaths. Though still somewhat limited, homeopathic educational opportunities in the United States are improving each year. The most rigorous form of training available is offered by weekend-based schools scattered throughout the country. Some of these schools accept only licensed practitioners; others are open to people of any background. A typical weekend-based school provides a three-year program of classes held one weekend per month. Courses cover homeopathic philosophy, materia medica, case-taking methodology, case analysis, and long-term patient management. Most schools require coursework in anatomy and physiology, as well as in pathology and disease. Classes are complemented by extensive homework and clinical training, where students sit in on patient interviews and case analysis with their instructors. Toward the end of their training, students begin to take on their own patients under the supervision of experienced homeopaths.

Another form of homeopathic training is attendance at workshops that cover an array of topics pertaining to homeopathic theory and practice. In fact, ongoing workshop attendance is required by all of the homeopathic certifying organizations. Some of these training events focus on particular remedies or groups of remedies. Others focus on the treatment of specific diseases or on a particular theoretical approach to case analysis and treatment. Using video recordings of patient interviews as well as "live cases" — patients who are treated by the lecturer at the workshop — workshops provide valuable learning experiences for beginning and advanced practitioners alike.

Finally, there are a number of intensive training courses (usually two-week courses) available. For example, each year the National Center for Homeopathy offers a two-week summer school that provides introductory classes for licensed practitioners, classes on veterinary homeopathy, and classes for lay people interested in learning more about self-care and homeopathic philosophy.

There is also the option to study abroad. A common destination is India, where homeopaths-in-training can apprentice themselves to master homeopaths at large clinics. Other aspiring homeopaths can train at schools in England, Scotland, Greece, or Germany. Some of the European schools offer high-quality correspondence programs. For example, I have been a student of the School of Homoeopathy in Devon, England, for several years. This school offers an intensive correspondence program for overseas students, complemented by clinical workshops held at various locations in the United States and Canada.

All in all, the availability of good homeopathic training in North America has improved dramatically in recent years. But it is still far from where it should be. In my opinion, homeopaths should try to rebuild the homeopathic educational system that was lost during the 20th century — full-time homeopathic medical schools that teach the basics of medicine alongside homeopathy, blended together in a harmonious way. The four-year schools that train naturopathic physicians provide a role model for this kind of institution. The product of such schools would be fully trained physicians who subscribe to the homeopathic, not allopathic, approach to disease. It may seem like a dream today, but it once was a reality — and can be again.

OTHER ISSUES: INSURANCE, ACCESS TO REMEDIES, AND RECOGNITION

Naturally, there are a host of other issues that must be addressed before homeopathy can assume its rightful place as a respected and widespread medical system in America. One is insurance. No medical treatment will become truly popular in the United States unless it is covered by health insurance. The primary hurdle will be winning coverage for treatment by unlicensed homeopaths. If the legality issue is resolved, insurance coverage will hopefully follow.

What about the tools of the homeopathic trade — the remedies? It is fortunate that the person who drafted the legislation that established the Food and Drug Administration in 1938 was a homeopath. New York Senator Royal Copeland, MD, embedded within that legislation assurances that the Homeopathic Pharmacopoeia of the United States (HPUS) would have formal legal standing. The Homeopathic Pharmacopoiea Convention of the United States (HPCUS) consists of pharmacists who meet several times each year to determine standards for the manufacture of approximately 1,350 homeopathic remedies in the HPUS. This body also serves as an intermediary between the homeopathic pharmaceutical industry and the government, ensuring that remedy manufacturing standards are upheld. There are currently around 10 homeopathic pharmaceutical companies operating in the United States, two of which have been in existence since the 1800s. An increasing number of mainstream companies are also beginning to manufacture and sell homeopathic remedies, especially combination remedies.

But are all remedies legal? Who can dispense them? Today, all remedies are nonprescription (i.e., they can be sold over-the-counter) as long as they are at dilutions that are nontoxic and they can be labeled as being indicated for a condition that is "self-limiting" — i.e., a condition that does not require medical diagnosis or monitoring. Labeled remedy indications must be based on provings in the homeopathic literature. Because of these restrictions, about 440 out of the 1,350 remedies in the

HPUS are prescription-only in low potencies (because of toxicity), while another 20 remedies are prescription-only in any potency.

There are also a few remedies that have dubious legal status, prescription or otherwise. Some have never been formally tested in a proving. Others are remedies for which precise manufacturing standards have never been formulated. Remedies made from illegal substances such as opium or cannabis also have questionable legal status, despite the fact that they are extremely important in clinical practice. Obviously, not a single molecule of drug matter is present in these remedies (not unless they are very low in potency). So why should they be illegal? In my view, all nontoxic remedies should be legal and freely available, though always used with caution and preferably under the guidance of a trained homeopath.

In the coming years, homeopathy must also seek to distinguish itself as a medical system. An important task will be one of definition: delineating what homeopathy is and what it is not, and educating the public and the medical establishment in that regard. For instance, homeopathy is not naturopathy or herbalism; nor is it simply the use of potentized remedies. Rather, homeopathy is the medical art that Samuel Hahnemann defined and developed: the treatment of the sick according to the Law of Similars.

But even after understanding and distinction and legality are won for homeopathy, credibility and advocacy will undoubtedly remain a challenge for many years to come. Hopefully, more medical studies like the ones described in Chapter 7 will dispel skepticism about homeopathy's effectiveness. Additional research on ultradilutions may convince mainstream scientists that the remedies do carry some kind of signature or information within them. And eventually, we may even discover how they work.

But the philosophical divide between the homeopathic and allopathic worlds will always remain. As long as allopathy relies on suppression as a primary therapeutic strategy, it will never be comfortable with the homeopathic message. Hopefully, just as people of different religions can learn to coexist, the landscape of American medicine can broaden to peacefully accommodate many different views and methods, even as they "agree to disagree."

OUR RIGHT TO HEALTH FREEDOM

Perhaps it is no accident that Minnesotans were able to legalize unlicensed health care in their state. Their strategy — asserting that legal alternative health care practice is a prerequisite to health freedom — resonates to the core of what America is all about. Why shouldn't we have the freedom to utilize the medicine of our choice? Why should particular medical practices be forced upon us, while others are forbidden? Shouldn't our bodies be as sacrosanct as our souls and our spirits? Shouldn't we have freedom of medicine in addition to freedom of religion and freedom of speech?

Truly, alternative medical systems like homeopathy should be embraced. The suppression of any kind of healing information may destroy our collective chances for survival on this planet — a planet that is becoming ever smaller and more populous. Boundaries are disappearing and diseases are spreading. Soon, diseases like tuberculosis may become commonplace in the United States once again. And with the increasing and indiscriminate use of antibiotics, stronger bacteria are developing. New mysterious viruses appear each year. Pollution is rampant. Food supplies are becoming compromised by drugs, toxic chemicals, and genetic engineering. Chronic disease has become almost the norm, even among our children. Global health crises are an increasing reality, biological warfare is a looming concern, and health care costs are skyrocketing.

It is becoming increasingly clear that new approaches to health care are desperately needed — approaches like homeopathy, which stress the importance of holistic and preventative approaches to disease and cure. Just as fostering peace is preferable to fomenting an arms race, cleaning up the environment and enhancing our natural defenses against disease are better strategies for achieving health than developing ever more potent and toxic drugs. This is what good homeopathic care can provide for us — a stronger and less susceptible vital force. And no matter what new disease does manage to come our way, homeopathy, at the very least, provides a means and a method for cure.

Its voice *must* be heard.

REFERENCES

[Albrecht] Albrecht, H., and A. Schutte, "Homeopathy Versus Antibiotics in Metaphylaxis of Infectious Diseases: A Clinical Study in Pig Fattening and Its Significance to Consumers," *Alternative Therapies*, Volume 5, Number 5, pp. 64–68 (September 1999).

[Alibeu] Alibeu, J. P., and J. Jobert, "Aconit en dilution homeopathique et agitation post-operatoire de l'enfant," *Pediatrie* (Bucur), 45:7–8, pp. 465–466 (1990).

[Bautista] Bautista, C., "American Women Homeopaths in WWI," *The American Homeopath*, Volume 4, page 139 (1998).

[Bellavite] Bellavite, Paolo, and Andrea Signorini, *The Emerging Science of Homeopathy: Complexity, Biodynamics, and Nanopharmacology*, North Atlantic Books, Berkeley, California (2002).

[Benveniste88] Davenas, E., F. Beauvais, J. Arnara, M. Oberbaum, B. Robinzon, A. Miadonna, A. Tedeschi, B. Pomeranz, P. Fortner, P. Belon, J. Sainte-Laudy, B. Poitevin, and J. Benveniste, "Human Basophil Degranulation Triggered by Very Dilute Antiserum Against IgE," *Nature*, Volume 333, Number 6176, pp. 816–818 (June 1988).

[Benveniste97] Aissa, J., P. Jurgens, W. Hsueh, and J. Benveniste, "Transatlantic Transfer of Digitized Antigen Signal by Telephone Link," *Journal of Allergy and Clinical Immunology*, 99:S175 (1997).

[Bohjalian] Bohjalian, Chris, *The Law of Similars*, Harmony Books, New York (1999).

[Bouchayer] Bouchayer, F., "Alternative Medicines: A General Approach to the French Situation," *Complementary Medical Research,* 4:4–8 (1990).

[Brennan] Brennan, Barbara Ann, *Hands of Light: A Guide to Healing Through the Human Energy Field*, Bantam Books, New York (1987).

[CalHealth] "Changes in the Population of Persons with Autism and Pervasive Developmental Disorders in California's Developmental Services System: 1987–1998," Report to the Legislature, Department of Developmental Services, California Health and Human Services Agency, 1600 Ninth Street, Room 240, Sacramento, CA 95814 (March 1, 1999).

[Castro] Castro, Miranda, *The Complete Homeopathy Handbook: A Guide to Everyday Health Care*, St. Martins Press, New York (1991).

[CastroNogueria] Castro, D., and G. Nogueria, "Use of the Nosode Meningococcinum As a Preventive Against Meningitis," *Journal of the American Institute for Homeopathy*, 68:211–219 (1975).

[Chopra] Chopra, Deepak, *Quantum Healing: Exploring the Frontiers of Mind Body Medicine,* Bantam Books, New York (1989).

[Clarke] Clarke, John Henry, *Life and Work of James Compton Burnett*, Homoeopathic Publishing Company, London (1904).

[Close] Close, Stuart, *The Genius of Homoeopathy*, Boericke and Tafel, Philadelphia, Pennsylvania (1924).

[Connelly] Connelly, Brian, "How Does Homeopathy Work?" *Homeopathy in Practice: Journal of the Alliance of Registered Homeopaths,* United Kingdom (March 2002). Also see: *home.attbi.com/~brc17/homeopathy0101.doc.*

[Coulter73] Coulter, Harris L., *Divided Legacy: The Conflict Between Homoeopathy and the American Medical Association, Volume III*, North Atlantic Books and Homeopathic Educational Services, Berkeley, California (1973).

[Coulter90] Coulter, Harris L., *Vaccination, Social Violence, and Criminality: The Medical Assault on the American Brain*, North Atlantic Books and Homeopathic Educational Services, Berkeley, California (1990).

[Coulter98] Coulter, Harris L., "The Paradigm Dispute in Medicine," *The American Homeopath*, Number 4, pp. 8–27 (1998).

[Daly] Daly, Joanna, "Revenge of the Deer: A Case of Androctonus," *The American Homeopath,* Volume 6, pp. 34–37 (2000).

[Dean] Dean, Michael Emmons, "A Homeopathic Origin for Placebo Controls," *Alternative Therapies,* Volume 6, Number 2, pp. 58–67 (March 2000).

[Eaton] Eaton, Charles Woodhull, "The Facts About Variolinum," in *Transactions of the American Institute of Homeopathy*, pp. 547–567 (1907).

[Eisenberg] Eisenberg, D. M., R. C. Kessler, C. Foster, F. E. Norlock, D. R. Calkins, and T. L. Delbanco, "Unconventional Medicine in the United States:

Prevalence, Costs, and Patterns of Use," *New England Journal of Medicine*, 328:4, pp. 246–252 (1993).

[Elia] Elia, Vittorio, and Marcella Nicolli, "Thermodynamics of Extremely Diluted Aqueous Solutions," *Annals of the New York Academy of Sciences*, 827, pp. 241–248 (June 1999).

[Ennis] Brown, V., and M. Ennis, "Flow-Cytometric Analysis of Basophil Activation: Inhibition by Histamine at Conventional and Homeopathic Concentrations," *Inflammation Research*, 50, Supplement(2), S47–S48 (2001).

[Evans] Evans, Linda Jane, "The 20th Century's Last Review of Homeopathy 101," *Homeopathy Today*, Volume 20, Number 2, pp. 9–10 (February 2000).

[Feingold] Feingold, Ben F., *Why Your Child Is Hyperactive,* Random House, New York (1985). Also see *www.feingold.org.*

[Ferley] Ferley, J. P., D. Zmirou, D. D'Adhemar, and F. Balducci, "A Controlled Evaluation of a Homeopathic Preparation in the Treatment of Influenza-Like Syndromes," *British Journal of Clinical Pharmacology*, 27, pp. 329–335 (1989).

[Filipponi] Filipponi, A., D. R. Bowron, C. Lobban, and J. L. Finney, *Physics Review Letters*, 79, p. 1293 (1997).

[Foubister] Foubister, D. M., "The Carcinosin Drug Picture," *British Homeopathic Journal*, 47, p. 201 (July 1958).

[Furtsch] Furtsch, T. A., "Some Notes on Avogadro's Number, 6.022×10^{23}," Tennessee Technological University, Cookeville, Tennessee, *gemini.tntech.edu/~tfurtsch/scihist/avogadro.htm.*

[Garcia-Swain] Garcia-Swain, Susan, "A Double-Blind, Placebo-Controlled Clinical Trial Applying Homeopathy to Chemical Dependency," Hahnemann College of Homeopathy, Albany, California (June 1993).

[GermanStudies] Participants in ongoing large-scale studies of homeopathy in Germany include: Claudia Witt and Stefan N. Willich, Institut Arbeits und Sozialmedizin, Universitetsklinikum Charite, Humboldt-Universite Berlin, Schumannstrasse 20–22, D-10098, Berlin, Germany; Harald Walach, Psychologisches Institut der Universitet Freiburg, D-79085, Freiburg, Germany; Max Haidvogl, Ludwig Boltzmann Institut fur Homeopathie, DeCrergasse 4, 8010, Graz, Austria; Marianne Heger, Research Center HomInt, P.O. Box 410240, D-76202, Karlsruhe, Germany; Michael Fischer,

Data Collection Center ClinWeb, Max-Planck-Strasse 2, 50858, Koln, Germany; and David Riley, Integrative Medicine Institute, P.O. Box 4310, Santa Fe, New Mexico 87502, USA.

[Gibson] Gibson et al., *Journal of Clinical Pharmacology*, 9, p. 453 (1980).

[Gordon] Gordon, Richard, *Quantum-Touch: The Power to Heal*, North Atlantic Books, Berkeley, California (1999).

[Gray] Gray, Bill, *Homeopathy: Science or Myth?*, North Atlantic Books and Homeopathic Educational Services, Berkeley, California (2000).

[Haehl] Haehl, R., *Samuel Hahnemann: His Life and Work*, translated from the German by M. Wheeler and W. Grundy, Volume 1, London (1931).

[Hahnemann] Hahnemann, Samuel, *Organon of the Medical Art (Sixth Edition)*, edited and annotated by Wenda Brewster O'Reilly, based on a translation by Stephen Decker, Birdcage Books, Redmond, Washington (1996).

[Hahnemann1stOrganon] Hahnemann, Samuel, *Organon Der Rationellen Heilkunde* (First Edition of the Organon), Arnoldischen Buchhandlung (1810).

[HahnemannCD] Hahnemann, Samuel, *The Chronic Diseases: Their Peculiar Nature and Their Homeopathic Cure*, Arnold, Dresden, Germany (1828). The second enlarged German edition of 1835 was translated by Prof. Louis H. Tafel, and is now published by B. Jain Publishers, New Delhi, India (1995).

[Haley] Haley, Boyd E., "Toxic Overload: Assessing the Role of Mercury in Autism," *Mothering*, Number 115, pp. 44–46 (November/December 2002).

[Handley] Handley, Rima, *A Homeopathic Love Story: The Story of Samuel and Melanie Hahnemann*, North Atlantic Books and Homeopathic Educational Services, Berkeley, California (1990).

[Hendersen] Hendersen, Charles W., "Are Journals Biased Against Alternative Medicine?" *World Disease Weekly*, Thomson Corporation Company, Birmingham, Alabama (April 9, 2000). Copyright 2000 by Charles W. Hendersen, IAC-ACC-NO 61209556.

[Herald] Reported in *The Sunday Herald*, "Autism Figures Soar in America" (January 6, 2002). Also see *www.sundayherald.com/21347*.

[Hershoff] Hershoff, Asa, "The Undiscovered Country," *Homeopathy Today*, Volume 20, Number 1, pp. 14–16 (January 2000).

[Herscu] Herscu, Paul, *Stramonium: With an Introduction to Analysis Using Cycles and Segments*, New England School of Homeopathy Press, Amherst, Massachusetts (1996).

[HerscuAut] Latchis, Spero, "Homeopathy and Autism: Report on a Presentation by Paul Herscu, ND, DHANP," *Homeopathy Today*, Volume 21, Number 10, pp. 20–21 (November 2001).

[Hoa] Hoa, J. Hui Bon, "Carcinosin: A Clinical and Pathogenetic Study," *The British Homoeopathic Journal* (July 1963).

[HomeopathyToday] *Homeopathy Today*, Volume 18, Number 7, p. 16 (July/August 1998).

[Hoover] Hoover, Todd, "Homeopathic Prophylaxis: Fact or Fiction," *Journal of the American Institute of Homeopathy* (Autumn 2001). Also see *www.homeopathyusa.org*.

[HoustonChronicle] "Caffeine May Fight Parkinson's Disease," *Houston Chronicle* (May 24, 2000). Also see Reuters News Service (May 23, 2000).

[Incao] Incao, Philip F., "How Vaccinations Work" (May 1999), *www.garynull.com/Documents/niin/how_vaccinations_work.htm*.

[India] "Indian Systems of Medicine Can Make HIV Patients Symptom Free," Indian Government Press Release (December 1, 1998). Reported in *Homeopathy Today*, Volume 19, Number 5, p. 6 (May 1999).

[Jacobs] Jacobs, Jennifer, L. Margarita Jimenez, Stephen S. Gloyd, James L. Gale, and Dean Crothers, "Treatment of Acute Childhood Diarrhea with Homeopathic Medicine: A Randomized Clinical Trial in Nicaragua," *Pediatrics*, Volume 93, Number 5, pp. 719–725 (May 1994).

[Jacobs00] Jacobs, J., L. M. Jimenez, M. D. Malthouse, E. Chapman, D. Crothers, M. Masuk, and W. B. Jonas, "Homeopathic Treatment of Acute Childhood Diarrhea: Results from a Clinical Trial in Nepal," *Journal of Alternative and Complementary Medicine*, Volume 6, pp. 131–139 (2000).

[Jacobs01] Jacobs, J., D. A. Springer, and D. Crothers, "Homeopathic Treatment of Acute Otitis Media in Children: A Preliminary Randomized

Placebo-Controlled Trial," *Pediatric Infectious Disease Journal*, 20, 2, pp. 177–183 (February 2001).

[JJonas] Jonas, Julian, "A Constitutional Case of Cantharis," unpublished paper (2000). Used with permission from the author via personal communication (May 2002).

[Jonas] Jonas, Wayne B., "Do Homeopathic Nosodes Protect Against Infection? An Experimental Test," *Alternative Therapies*, Volume 5, Number 5, pp. 36–40 (September 1999).

[Jonas01] Jonas, Wayne B., "Directions for Research in Complementary Medicine and Bioterrorism," *Alternative Therapies*, Volume 8, Number 2, pp. 30–31 (March/April 2002). Originally presented as testimony before the U.S. House Committee on Government Reform, "Comprehensive Medical Care for Bioterrorism Exposure: Are We Making Evidence-Based Decisions? What Are the Research Needs?" (November 14, 2001).

[Jonas&Jacobs] Jonas, Wayne B., and Jennifer Jacobs, *Healing with Homeopathy*, Warner, New York (1996).

[Jongma] Jongma, Rienk T., Yuhui Huang, Shimning Shi, and Alec M. Wodtke, "Rapid Evaporative Cooling Suppresses Fragmentation in Mass Spectrometry: Synthesis of 'Unprotonated' Water Cluster Ions," *J. Phys. Chemistry A*, 102, pp. 8847–8854 (1998).

[Kaufman] Kaufman, Martin, *Homeopathy in America: The Rise and Fall of a Medical Heresy*, Johns Hopkins Press, Baltimore, Maryland (1971).

[KaufmanD] Kaufman, David W., Judith P. Kelly, Lynn Rosenberg, Theresa E. Anderson, Allen A. Mitchell, "Recent Patterns of Medication Use in the Ambulatory Adult Population of the United States," *Journal of the American Medical Association (JAMA)*, Volume 287, Number 3, pp. 337–344 (January 16, 2002).

[Kent] Kent, James Tyler, *Lectures on Homoeopathic Philosophy*, North Atlantic Books and Homeopathic Educational Services, Berkeley, California (1979). First published by Examiner Printing House, Lancaster, Pennsylvania (1900).

[KentRep] Kent, James Tyler, *Repertory of the Homoeopathic Materia Medica*, Sixth American Edition, B. Jain Publishers Pvt. Ltd., New Delhi, 110 055 (reprinted 1995). The first edition was originally published by Examiner Printing House, Lancaster, Pennsylvania (1897).

[Kessler] Kessler, R. C., R. B. Davis, D. F. Foster, M. I. Van Rompay, E. E. Walters, S. A. Wilkey, T. J. Kaptchuk, and D. M. Eisenberg, "Long-Term Trends in the Use of Complementary and Alternative Medical Therapies in the United States," *Annals of Internal Medicine*, 135, pp. 262–268 (2001).

[Kleijnen] Kleijnen, J., P. Knipschild, and G. ter Riet, "Clinical Trials of Homeopathy," *British Medical Journal*, 302:316–323 (1991).

[Knerr] Knerr, Calvin B., *Life of Hering*, Magee Press, Philadelphia, Pennsylvania (1940).

[Lansky] Lansky, Amy L., "Max's Story: A Carcinosin Cure," *Homeopathy Online*, Issue 5, (January 1998), *www.lyghtforce.com/HomeopathyOnline/Issue5*. Also see *www.renresearch.com/autism.html*. A condensed version of this article appeared in *Similia, Publication of the Australian Homoeopathic Association*, Volume 11, Number 2, pp. 29–35 (July 1998).

[Lasser] Lasser, Karen E., Paul D. Allen, Steffie J. Woolhandler, David U. Himmelstein, Sidney M. Wolfe, David H. Bor, "Timing of New Black Box Warnings and Withdrawals for Prescription Medications," *Journal of the American Medical Association (JAMA)*, 287 (17), pp. 2215–2220 (May 2002).

[Lazarou] Lazarou, J., B. H. Pomeranz, P. N. Corey, "Incidence of Adverse Drug Reactions in Hospitalized Patients: A Meta-Analysis of Prospective Studies," *Journal of the American Medical Association (JAMA)*, 279 (15), pp. 1200–1205 (April 1998).

[Lewith] Lewith, George, "The Homeopathic Conundrum Revisited," *Alternative Therapies*, Volume 5, Number 5, p. 32 (September 1999).

[Linde] Linde, K., N. Clausius, G. Ramirez, D. Melchart, F. Eitel, L. Hedges, and W. Jonas, "Are the Clinical Effects of Homoeopathy Placebo Effects? A Meta-Analysis of Placebo-Controlled Trials," *The Lancet*, Volume 250, pp. 834–843 (September 20, 1997).

[Maiolino] Maiolino, Ramona, "A Miraculous Case," *Homeopathy Today*, Volume 15, Number 11 (December 1995).

[Melnychuk] Melnychuk, John D., "A Case of Germanium," *The American Homeopath*, Volume 6, pp. 121–124 (2000).

[Mercola] Mercola, Joseph M., "Vaccine Insanity," *The Mercola Newsletter* (February 2, 2000), *www.mercola.com/2002/feb/2/vaccine_insanity.htm*.

[Milgrom] Milgrom, Lionel, "Experiments Have Backed What Was Once a Scientific 'Heresy,' says Lionel Milgrom," *Guardian Weekly* (March 15, 2001).

[Minnesota] *Complementary Medicine: Final Report to the Legislature*, Minnesota Department of Health, Health Economics Program (January 15, 1998), *www.health.state.mn.us/divs/hpsc/ hep/reports/compmed.pdf*.

[Moher] Moher, David, et. al., "Does Quality of Reports of Randomised Trials Affect Estimates of Intervention Efficacy Reported in Meta-Analyses?" *The Lancet*, Volume 352, Issue 9, 128, p. 609 (1998).

[Muscat] Muscat, Michael, "Homeopathy Study Confirms Biological Action of Ultra-High Dilutions," *Alternative Therapies*, Volume 5, Number 5, p. 26 (September 1999).

[Neustaedter] Neustaedter, Randall, *The Vaccine Guide: Making an Informed Choice*, North Atlantic Books and Homeopathic Educational Services, Berkeley, California (1996).

[NYTimes] Eichenwald, Kurt, and Gina Kolata, "Drug Trials Hide Conflicts for Doctors: Research for Hire," *The New York Times* (May 16, 1999).

[OTA] "Assessing the Efficacy and Safety of Medical Technologies," Congressional Office of Technology Assessment, Washington, D.C. (1978:7).

[Panos] Panos, Maesimund B., and Jane Heimlich, *Homeopathic Medicine at Home: Natural Remedies for Everyday Ailments and Minor Injuries*, J. P. Tarcher, Los Angeles, California (1980).

[Papp] Papp, R., G. Schuback, E. Beck, et al., "Oscillococcinum(R) in Patients with Influenza-Like Syndromes: A Placebo-Controlled Double-Blind Evaluation," *British Homeopathic Journal,* 87, pp. 69–76 (1998).

[Parish] Parish, C. R., "The Relationship Between Humoral and Cell-Mediated Immunity," *Transplant. Rev.* 13 (1972:3).

[Perko] Perko, Sandra, *The Homeopathic Treatment of Influenza: Surviving Influenza Epidemics and Pandemics Past, Present, and Future with Homeopathy*, Benchmark Homeopathic Publications, San Antonio, Texas (1999).

[Phatak] Phatak, S. R., *Materia Medica of Homeopathic Medicines*, Indian Books and Periodicals Syndicate, New Delhi 110 005, India (1977).

[Pieterse] "Zola Makes a Stunning Comeback," News24.com, South African Press Association (December 29, 2001), *www.news24.com/News24/Sport/Athletics/0,1231,2-9-28_1125482,00.html.*

[Poitevin] Poitevin, B., "Integrating Homoeopathy in Health Systems," *Bulletin of the World Health Organization*, 77(2), pp. 160–166 (1999).

[Provencal] Provencal, R. A., K. Roth, J. B. Paul, C. N. Chapo, R. N. Casaes, R. J. Saykally, G. S. Tschumper, and H. F. Schaefer, III, "Hydrogen Bonding in Alcohol Clusters: A Comparative Study by Infrared Cavity Ringdown Laser Absorption Spectroscopy," *J. Phys. Chem. A*, 104, 1423 (2000).

[Provings] "Hahnemann's Provings," collected by W. Taylor, edited and annotated by A. L. Lansky, *The American Homeopath*, Volume 6, p. 74 (2000).

[Radin] Radin, Dean, *The Conscious Universe*, Harper Collins, New York (1997).

[Ramakrishan] Ramakrishnan, A. U. and Catherine R. Coulter, *A Homoeopathic Approach to Cancer*, Quality Medical Publishing, St. Louis, Missouri, pp. 67–68 (2001).

[Rastogi] Rastogi, D. P., V. P. Singh, V. Singh, S. K. Dey, and K. Rao, "Homeopathy in HIV Infection: Trial Report of a Double-Blind Placebo-Controlled Study," *British Homeopathic Journal*, Volume 88, Number 2 (April 1999).

[Reichenberg-Ullman95] Reichenberg-Ullman, Judyth, "A Homeopathic Approach to Behavioral Problems," *Mothering*, Number 74, pp. 97–101 (Spring 1995).

[Reichenberg-Ullman96] Reichenberg-Ullman, Judyth, and Robert Ullman, *Ritalin-Free Kids: Safe and Effective Homeopathic Medicine for ADD and Other Behavioral and Learning Problems*, Prima Publishing, Rocklin, California (1996).

[Reichenberg-Ullman04] Reichenberg-Ullman, Judyth, Robert Ullman, and Ian Luepker, *A Drug-Free Approach to Autism and Asperger's: Homeopathic Care for Exceptional Kids*, Starfish Specialty Press, Higganum, Connecticut (2004).

[Reilly94] Reilly, D., M. Taylor, N. Beattie, et al., "Is Evidence for Homoe-opathy Reproducible?" *Lancet*, 344, p. 1601–1606 (December 10, 1994).

[Reilly00] Taylor, Morag A., David Reilly, Robert H. Llewellyn-Jones, Charles McSharry, and Tom C. Aitchison, "Randomised Controlled Trial of

Homoeopathy Versus Placebo in Perennial Allergic Rhinitis with Overview of Four Trial Series," *British Medical Journal (BMJ)*, 321, pp. 471–476 (August 19, 2000).

[Resch] Resch, G., and V. Gutmann, *Scientific Foundations of Homeopathy*, Barthel and Barthel Publishing, Berg am Starnberger, Germany (1987).

[Roberts] Roberts, Herbert A., *The Principles and Art of Cure by Homoeopathy*, B. Jain Publishers, New Delhi, India (1995). First published by Homoeopathic Publishing Company (1936).

[Rosenstock] Rosenstock, Linda, "Special Interests Undermine Objectivity of Scientific Research," *American Journal of Public Health*, Volume 92, pp. 14–18 (January 2002).

[Ross] Ross, Melanie F., "University of Florida Researchers Cite Possible Link Between Autism, Schizophrenia and Diet," University of Florida Press Release, reported in *Science Daily* (March 16, 1999), *www.sciencedaily.com/releases/1999/03/990316103010.htm*.

[Rush] Rush, Benjamin. For more information on Benjamin Rush, MD, see "Benjamin Rush, MD, A Bibliographic Guide," compiled by Claire G. Fox, Gordon L. Miller, and Jacquelyn C. Miller, *American History, Bibliographies and Indexes*, No. 31, Greenwood Press, Westport, Connecticut (1996).

[Sankaran] Sankaran, Rajan, *The Spirit of Homoeopathy*, Homoeopathic Medical Publishers, Bombay, India (1992).

[Sankaran97] Sankaran, Rajan, *The Soul of Remedies*, Homoeopathic Medical Publishers, Bombay, India (1997).

[Sarno] Sarno, John, *Mind over Back Pain: A Radically New Approach to the Diagnosis and Treatment of Back Pain*, Mass Market Paperback, Berkley Publishing Group, New York (1986).

[Scholten] Scholten, Jan, *Homoeopathy and the Elements*, Stichting Alonnissos, Utrecht, The Netherlands (1996).

[Sheldrake] Sheldrake, Rupert, *The Presence of the Past: Morphic Resonance and the Habits of Nature*, Park Street Press, Rochester, Vermont (1988).

[Shinohara] Shinohara, H., N. Nishis, and N. Washida, *J. Chem. Phys*, 84, 5561 (1986).

[Singh] Singh, V. K., S. X. Lin, and V. C. Yang, "Serological Association of Measles Virus and Human Herpes Virus-6 with Brain Autoantibodies in Autism," *Clinical Immunological Immunopathology*, 89:105–108 (1998).

[Sloan] Sloan, E. D., Jr., and F. Fleyfel, *Ind. Chemical Engineering Journal*, 37, 1281 (1991).

[Spranger] Spranger, J., "Testing the Effectiveness of Homeopathic and Antibiotic Medication in the Frame of Herd Reorganisation of Sub-Clinical Mastitis in Milk Cows," *British Homeopathic Journal,* 89 (suppl. 1): S62 (2000).

[Starfield] Starfield, Barbara, "Is U.S. Health Really the Best in the World?" *Journal of the American Medical Association (JAMA)*, 284(4), pp. 483–485 (July 2000).

[Stein] Stein, Diane, *Essential Reiki: A Complete Guide to an Ancient Healing Art,* The Crossing Press, Santa Cruz, California (1995).

[Sun1] Sun, Zhongjie, J. Robert Cade, Melvin J. Fregly, and R. Malcolm Privette, "Beta-Casomorphin Induces Fos-Like Immunoreactivity in Discrete Brain Regions Relevant to Schizophrenia and Autism," *Autism: The International Journal of Research and Practice,* Volume 3, Number 1, pp. 67–83 (March 1999).

[Sun2] Sun, Zhongjie, and J. Robert Cade, "A Peptide Found in Schizophrenia and Autism Causes Behavioral Changes in Rats," *Autism: The International Journal of Research and Practice,* Volume 3, Number 1, pp. 85–95 (March 1999).

[Targ] Targ, Elizabeth, "Distant Healing," *IONS Noetic Sciences Review*, Number 49, pp. 24–29 (August–November 1999).

[Traub] Traub, Michael, "Homeopathic Prophylaxis," *Journal of Naturopathic Medicine,* Volume 5, Number 1, pp. 50–61 (1994). For full text on the Iowa case, see *www.homeopathic.co.nz/AIH/smallpox1.htm.*

[Upcher] Upcher, Canon Roland, "Consumption and Vaccination," letter to *The Homoeopathic World* (September 1924).

[Uppsala] "Free Clusters: From the Isolated Atom to the Infinite Solid," Department of Physics, Uppsala Universitet, *fysik5.fysik.uu.se/jobs/clusters.html#source.*

[USAToday] Cauchon, Dennis, "FDA Advisers Tied to Industry," *USA Today* (September 25, 2000).

[Vermeulen] Vermeulen, Frans, *Synoptic Materia Medica 2*, Merlijn Publishers, Haarlem, The Netherlands (1996).

[Vithoulkas] Vithoulkas, George, *The Science of Homeopathy*, Grove Press, New York (1980).

[Vithoulkas79] Vithoulkas, George, *Homeopathy: Medicine of the New Man*, Fireside, Simon & Schuster, New York (1979).

[Viza] Viza, Dimitri, "From Placebo to Homeopathy: The Fear of the Irrational," *The Scientist*, Volume 12, Number 18 (September 14, 1998).

[Wakefield] Wakefield, Andrew, et al., "Ileal-Lymphoid-Nodular Hyperplasia, Non-Specific Colitis, and Pervasive Developmental Disorder in Children," *Lancet*, 351, pp. 637–641 (1998).

[Watson] Watson, Ian, *A Guide to the Methodologies of Homoeopathy*, Cutting Edge Publications, Kendal, Cumbria, England (1999).

[Wharton] Wharton, R., and G. Lewith, "Complementary Medicine and the General Practitioner," *British Medical Journal*, 292, pp. 1490–1500 (1986).

[White] White, Patti, "Hepatitis B Vaccine: A School Nursing Perspective for the Congressional Hearings on May 18, 1999, Regarding the Safety of the Hepatitis B Vaccine that Is Being Mandated for Newborns and Now Older Children in America," Statement to the Subcommittee on Criminal Justice, Drug Policy, and Human Resources of the Committee on Government Reform, U.S. House of Representatives, *www.alternativeparenting.com/health/HepB.asp*.

[Whitmont] Whitmont, Edward C., *Psyche and Substance*, North Atlantic Books and Homeopathic Educational Services, Berkeley, California (1991).

[Wilson] Wilson, Harold J., "Specific High-Potency Homeopathic Remedies for Heavy Metal Poisoning," *The Layman Speaks*, p. 163 (June 1978).

[Winston] Winston, Julian, *The Faces of Homoeopathy*, Great Auk Publishing, Tawa, New Zealand (1999).

E-mail Citations

The following citations are for communications taken from an international homeopathy mailing list: *homeopathy@homeolist.com*. Each citation gives the name and city of the contributor (unless they have requested anonymity) and the month in which the contribution was made. All citations, including anonymous citations, appear with the explicit permission of the author. To find out more about this mailing list, visit *www.homeopathyhome.com/web/descriptions/homlist.shtml.*

[Anon1] Anonymous, 4-1998.

[Anon2] Anonymous, 12-1998.

[AS] Anna Strong, Farmington Hills, Michigan, 11-1999.

[CG] Charlotte Garland, Winnsboro, Texas, 12-1998.

[CK] Christian Kurz, Eisenstadt, Austria, 12-1997

[DK] David Kempson, Brisbane, Australia, 10-2000.

[DL1] David Little, Dalhousie, India, 3-2000.

[DL2] David Little, Dalhousie, India, 7-1999.

[FT] Francis Treuherz, London, England, 2-1998.

[GE] Gini Ellis, Cupertino, California, 12-1998.

[GP] Gopal Pandey, Matthews-Charlotte, North Carolina, 6-2000.

[JS] John Summerville, Mangonui, New Zealand, 6-2000.

[LJ] Linda Jarosiewicz, Montreal, Quebec, Canada, 6-2000.

[MB] Marybeth Buchele-Moseman, Menomonie, Wisconsin, 11-2000.

[MBohle1] Maria Bohle, Egg Harbor Township, New Jersey, 1-1999.

[MBohle2] Maria Bohle, Egg Harbor Township, New Jersey, 12-1999.

[MC] Muhammed R. K. Chishty, Chicago, Illinois, 10-1999.

[MK] Martha Kovacs, Brampton, Ontario, Canada, 4-1999.

[MM] Mary Marlowe, Athens, Georgia, 12-1998.

[MW] Mary Wisner, writer and editor, mary@marywisner.com, 11-1997.

[RM] Ron Meek, Awanui, New Zealand, 8-1998.

[SD] Shonit Danwer, Blacktown, New South Wales, Australia, 2-2000.

[SL1] Spero Latchis, Brattleboro, Vermont, 11-1998.

[SL2] Spero Latchis, Brattleboro, Vermont, 1-1999.

[SN] Sheri Nakken, Wales, United Kingdom, 2-1998 and 3-1998.

[SO] Suriya Osman, Melaka, Malaysia, 9-1998

[SW1] Steve Waldstein, Aurora, Colorado, 8-1997

[SW2] Steve Waldstein, Aurora, Colorado, 6-1998

[VCD] Virginia Downey, Lakewood, New Jersey, 7-1997.

[WT1] Will Taylor, Portland, Oregon, 2-1998

[WT2] Will Taylor, Portland, Oregon, 6-1999

[WT3] Will Taylor, Portland, Oregon, 2-1998

[WT4] Will Taylor, Portland, Oregon, 3-1997.

[WT5] Will Taylor, Portland, Oregon, 3-1999.

SUGGESTED READING

The best source of books on homeopathy are the homeopathic booksellers. The two largest in the United States are *Minimum Price Books*, which carries just about every book on homeopathy, as well as tapes and software (*www.minimum.com*, 1-800-663-8272), and *Homeopathic Educational Services*, which sells book, tapes, software, and remedies, and serves as a publisher of many books on homeopathy and other forms of alternative health care (*www.homeopathic.com*, 1-800-359-9051).

Self-Help Books

- Castro, Miranda, *The Complete Homeopathy Handbook: A Guide to Everyday Health Care*, St. Martins Press (1991).

- Castro, Miranda, *Homeopathy for Pregnancy, Birth and Your Baby's First Year,* St. Martins Press (1997).

- Cummings, Stephen, and Dana Ullman, *Everybody's Guide to Homeopathic Medicines: Safe and Effective Medicines for You and Your Family*, 3rd Revised Edition, J. P. Tarcher, Los Angeles (1997).

- Lockie, Andrew, *The Family Guide To Homoeopathy*, Fireside (1993).

- Panos, Maesimund B., and Jane Heimlich, *Homeopathic Medicine at Home: Natural Remedies for Everyday Ailments and Minor Injuries,* J. P. Tarcher, Los Angeles (1980).

- Reichenberg-Ullman, Judyth, and Robert Ullman, *Homeopathic Self Care: The Quick and Easy Guide for the Whole Family*, Prima Publishing, Rocklin, California (1997).

- Reichenberg-Ullman, Judyth, and Robert Ullman, *Whole Woman Homeopathy: The Comprehensive Guide to Treating PMS, Menopause, Cystitis, and Other Problems Naturally and Effectively,* Prima Publishing, Rocklin, California (2000).

- Ullman, Dana, *Homeopathic Medicine for Children and Infants,* J.P. Tarcher, Los Angeles (1992).

Patient Education

- Dooley, Timothy, *Homeopathy: Beyond Flat Earth Medicine*, Timing Publications, San Diego, California (1995).

- Reichenberg-Ullman, Judyth, and Robert Ullman, *The Patient's Guide to Homeopathic Medicine,* Picnic Point Press (1995).

- Reichenberg-Ullman, Judyth, and Robert Ullman, *Prozac-Free — Homeopathic Medicine for Depression, Anxiety, and Other Mental and Emotional Problems,* Prima Publishing, Rocklin, California (1999).

- Reichenberg-Ullman, Judyth, and Robert Ullman, *Rage Free Kids — Homeopathic Medicine for Defiant, Aggressive, and Violent Children,* Prima Publishing, Rocklin, California (1999).

- Reichenberg-Ullman, Judyth, and Robert Ullman, *Ritalin Free Kids — Safe and Effective Homeopathic Medicine for ADD and Other Behavioral and Learning Problems,* Prima Publishing, Rocklin, California (1996).

- Reichenberg-Ullman, Judyth, Robert Ullman, and Ian Luepker, *A Drug-Free Approach to Autism and Asperger's: Homeopathic Care for Exceptional Kids,* Starfish Specialty Press, Higganum, Connecticut (2004).

- Ullman, Dana, *Discovering Homeopathy — Your Introduction To the Science and Art of Homeopathic Medicine,* North Atlantic Books (1991).

Research

- Bellavite, Paolo, and Andrea Signorini, *The Emerging Science of Homeopathy: Complexity, Biodynamics, and Nanopharmacology*, North Atlantic Books, Berkeley, California (2002).

- Gray, Bill, *Homeopathy: Science or Myth?*, North Atlantic Books and Homeopathic Educational Services, Berkeley, California (2000).

- Jonas, Wayne B., and Jennifer Jacobs, *Healing with Homeopathy*, Warner, New York (1996).

Philosophy

- Close, Stuart, *The Genius of Homoeopathy: Lectures and Essays on Homoeopathic Philosophy*, Boericke and Tafel (1924). Now printed by B. Jain Publishers, New Delhi, India (1993).

- Hahnemann, Samuel, *Organon of the Medical Art,* edited and annotated by Wenda Brewster O'Reilly, Birdcage Books, Redmond, Washington (1996).

- Kent, James Tyler, *Lectures on Homoeopathic Philosophy*, North Atlantic Books and Homeopathic Educational Services, Berkeley, California (1979). First published by Examiner Printing House, Lancaster, Pennsylvania (1900).

- Vithoulkas, George, *The Science of Homeopathy*, Grove Press, New York (1980).

- Whitmont, Edward C., *Psyche and Substance,* North Atlantic Books and Homeopathic Educational Services, Berkeley, California (1991)

History

- Coulter, Harris L., *Divided Legacy: The Conflict Between Homoeopathy and the American Medical Association*, North Atlantic Books and Homeopathic Educational Services, Berkeley, California (1973)

- Handley, Rima, *A Homeopathic Love Story: The Story of Samuel and Melanie Hahnemann*, North Atlantic Books and Homeopathic Educational Services, Berkeley, California (1990).

- Winston, Julian, *The Faces of Homoeopathy,* Great Auk Publishing, Tawa, New Zealand (1999).

Vaccination

- Coulter, Harris L., *Vaccination, Social Violence, and Criminality: The Medical Assault on the American Brain*, North Atlantic Books and Homeopathic Educational Services, Berkeley, California (1990).

- Miller, Neil Z., *Vaccines: Are They Really Safe and Effective? A Parent's Guide to Childhood Shots*, 10th Updated and Revised Edition, New Atlantean Press (2001).

- Neustaedter, Randall, *The Vaccine Guide: Making an Informed Choice*, North Atlantic Books and Homeopathic Educational Services, Berkeley, California (1996).

HELPFUL RESOURCES

HOMEOPATHIC ORGANIZATIONS

National Center for Homeopathy (NCH)

The main organization representing the homeopathic consumer in the United States, the NCH publishes an excellent monthly magazine, *Homeopathy Today*. The NCH also holds a yearly conference each spring, open to the public, as well as a two-week summer school.

National Center for Homeopathy
801 North Fairfax Street, Suite 306
Alexandria, Virginia 22314
877-624-0613 (toll free)
info@homeopathic.org
www.homeopathic.org

North American Society of Homeopaths (NASH)

This professional organization represents all certified homeopaths in North America. NASH publishes a yearly journal, *The American Homeopath*, and also holds a yearly conference each fall.

North American Society of Homeopaths
1122 East Pike Street #1122
Seattle, Washington 98122
206-720-7000
nashinfo@aol.com
www.homeopathy.org

Homeopathic Academy of Naturopathic Physicians (HANP)

This organization represents naturopaths who specialize in homeopathy. The HANP publishes a journal, *Simillimum*, and also holds a yearly case conference.

Homeopathic Academy for Naturopathic Physicians
1412 W. Washington Street
Boise, Idaho 83702
208-336-3390
info@hanp.net
www.hanp.net

Council for Homeopathic Certification (CHC)
This organization certifies classical homeopaths in the United States and
Canada.

> Council for Homeopathic Certification
> PMB 187
> 17051 SE 272nd Street, Suite #43
> Covington, Washington 98042
> 866-242-3399 (toll free)
> chcinfo@homeopathicdirectory.com
> *www.homeopathicdirectory.com*

USEFUL HOMEOPATHY WEB SITES

- *www.homeopathyhome.com* — A comprehensive homeopathy site that can be used to find all others. For example, if you click on Directory, you will be led to country-specific practitioner lists.

- *www.homeopathicdirectory.com* — Referrals to all certified homeopaths in the United States and Canada.

- *www.homeopathy-cures.com/html/referrals_to_homeopaths.html* — Another referral list to recommended classical homeopaths in the United States and Canada.

- *www.minimum.com* — Minimum Price Books. A good place to order homeopathic books, tapes, software, etc. This site also has book reviews, as well as a comprehensive list of *homeopathic educational facilities.*

- *www.homeopathic.com* — Homeopathic Educational Services. Another great place to buy homeopathic books, tapes, software, medicines, and courses.

VACCINATION INFORMATION SITES

- National Vaccine Information Center: *www.909shot.com*

- Think Twice Global Vaccine Institute: *www.thinktwice.com*

- Well Within: *www.nccn.net/~wwithin/vaccine.htm*

HEALTH FREEDOM WEB SITES

- National Health Freedom Coalition: *www.nationalhealthfreedom.org*
  This site includes pointers to all of the state health freedom web sites, including the sites listed below.

- California — California Health Freedom Coalition: *www.californiahealthfreedom.org*

- Florida -- Florida Health Freedom Action *www.floridahealthfreedom.org*

- Georgia — Complementary and Alternative Medicine Association: *www.camaweb.org*

- Minnesota — Minnesota Natural Health Coalition: *www.minnesotanaturalhealth.org*

- Massachusetts -- Health Freedom Massachusetts *www.healthfreedommassachusetts.org*

- New Jersey — New Jersey Natural Health Coalition: *www.njnhc.org*

- New York — New York Natural Health Project: *www.nynaturalhealthproject.org*

- Oklahoma — Health Freedom Action Network: *www.oklahomahealthfreedom.org*

- Rhode Island — Coalition for Natural Health: *www.naturalhealth.org*

IMPOSSIBLE CURE WEB SITE: *www.impossiblecure.com*

Check this site for information about ordering additional copies of *Impossible Cure* (including bulk discounts) and for ongoing updates on the information provided in this book. The *Impossible Cure* site also includes a database facility that enables readers to share their own stories of homeopathic cure.

INDEX

S

ABOUT THE AUTHOR

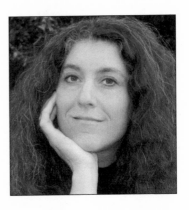

Amy Lansky grew up in a suburb of Buffalo, New York. She graduated from the University of Rochester in 1977 with degrees in mathematics and computer science, and she received her doctorate in computer science from Stanford University in 1983. After several years working at various Silicon Valley research institutions (including SRI International, NASA Ames Research Center, and three years as a consulting associate professor at Stanford), Lansky made an unusual career move: she became a student, writer, promoter, and, most recently, practitioner of homeopathic medicine. This was prompted by the miraculous cure of her son's autism with homeopathy. She is dedicated to helping others — especially families with autistic children — discover the curative powers of homeopathy.

Lansky's homeopathic studies have included foundational course work with Misha Norland's School of Homoeopathy in Devon, England; completion of the Homeopathic Master Clinician's course with Louis Klein; and studies with Simon Taffler, Sadhna Thakkar, Jan Scholten, and Alize Timmerman. For two years she served as coeditor of *The American Homeopath*, the journal of the North American Society of Homeopaths. Lansky is also an executive board member of the California Health Freedom Coalition, the organization that sponsored SB-577, the California health freedom bill that was passed in September 2002. In 2003 she became a board member of the National Center for Homeopathy, based in Alexandria, Virginia.

Lansky lives in the San Francisco Bay Area with her husband Steve Rubin and her two sons, Izaak and Max Rubin. An avid amateur musician, she has been a vocalist in several local rock bands and has studied piano composition and improvisation. In addition to music and homeopathy, she enjoys painting, needlework, swimming, and canoeing the lakes of Canada.